Mercy
A Second Chance

By Ebb Galvin

The cover photo is a brass relief of Catherine McAuley, founder of the Sisters of Mercy, created by artist Marie Henderson, RSM, also a Sister of Mercy.

ISBN: 1492100617
ISBN 13: 9781492100614
Library of Congress Control Number: 2013914880
LCCN Imprint Name: CreateSpace Independent Publishing
Platform, North Charleston, SC

This book is dedicated to
Lisa, my wife and best friend,
and Doctor Armando Sardi, my bowling buddy.

Contents

Prologue

My wife Lisa had had a decent life so far—a pretty good job, as jobs go; a devoted family, pets included; a circle of trusted local buddies; and a further network of lifelong friends and extended family. Lately she had been feeling bloated, then nauseous as well. In fact she had felt increasingly listless for months if not years. She called her doctor, who sent for an ultrasound: ascites, excess fluid in the abdominal cavity.

Next was a CT scan, which provided a horizontal view of the interior of the abdomen. Lisa assumed her doctor would call her in timely fashion, and when she didn't, she felt very anxious. Nor were her calls returned. She then called her gynecologist, Doctor Marcella Roenneburg, who had been a friend of the family even before Lisa had begun to see her as a patient. Would Marcy intervene on her behalf?

It was early August. Lisa arrived home from work one late afternoon, and a summer breeze stirred the maple leaves on the cluster of trees in our front yard, causing their shadows on the maroon brick of our modest row home to swell and recede, as though breathing.

Marcy called. Having seen the CT scan, she was almost certain Lisa had cancer and was prepared to recommend a consultation with Dr. Armando Sardi at Mercy Medical Center in Baltimore, only a short drive away, a visit that occurred two days later.

Lisa was diagnosed with a cancer--peritoneal carcinomatosis--and her initial web search turned up a dire prognosis, with the natural history of the disease, observed in untreated patients, leaving her about three or four months to live.

Lisa was no longer anxious, but terrified. A crucial part of her life was her devotion to our sole child, Danny, who was about to enter his senior year of college. The idea that she would be cheated of seeing the fruition of her efforts in nurturing him all those years was unbearable, and she spilled her heart to Marcy.

Marcy was quick to offer support: "Fight this thing head-on, take one day at a time, do everything Doctor Sardi tells you, and you'll see Danny go on to do great things."

One

For extreme diseases, extreme methods of cure…
are most suitable. --from Hippocrates's Aphorisms

Many of the things that plague us come from outside our bodies. Our bodies generally recognize these things as intruders, and our immune system, led by various types of white blood cells, attacks them. If our body is overwhelmed, or if we wish to speed up the healing process, we can take antibiotics, which kill harmful bacteria but are usually safe for our own cells. We also have benefited from vaccines and treatments that cure what would have killed our ancestors; in the last century, the lifespan of the average American has jumped from forty-seven years to seventy-eight years. A vaccine was developed for diphtheria in 1913, for example, and its widespread use increased after the 1925 *Great Race of Mercy,* when dogsleds carried the vaccine to Nome, Alaska. Malaria and tetanus, among many other diseases, are now rare. Smallpox has been eradicated, with only trace amounts kept in labs, for one reason or another.

But cancer is different. Cancer is our own cells gone rogue.

Our body comprises trillions of cells, including more than two hundred different types of cells, and the life of each individual cell is in many ways analogous to a beehive, or an ant colony, or even the entire body itself, at least in terms of function. In the middle of the cell is the nucleus, which carries the entire genome, twenty-three pairs of chromosomes, which collectively contains all our genes. Though almost all those genes are the same from person to person, and even to a lesser extent from species to species, the small differences that do exist are what make each person unique. The nucleus controls much of the other activity in the cell, and when the cell splits in half through the process of meiosis, the split begins in the nucleus.

Outside the nucleus is the cytoplasm, which contains organelles, tiny organs within the cell, such as mitochondria, lysosomes, and the Golgi apparatus, as well as the endomembrane system. All this moves water, oxygen, and nutrients around the cell and creates proteins and enzymes, many of which are necessary for growth, reproduction, and cell function. Middle school biology, for those who don't later go into medicine.

Like the beehive or the ant colony, normally everything is functional.

Almost all types of cells replicate, and that is usually a good thing. A pathologist can look at samples under a microscope: Here are blood cells, all alike. Here are bone cells, all alike. But when the cells look different, they can be cancer. Cancer results from damaged chromosomes.

Though some *tumors* are benign, with no threat of invading surrounding space, all *cancer* is malignant. Some malignant cancer is *in situ*, which means it hasn't spread yet to the surrounding space, while some is *invasive*. Cancer can be solid, such as a growth on an organ, or hematological, such as leukemia, which is the uncontrolled replication of white blood cells. Left untreated, cancer will continue to grow, and treatment options almost always need to be explored.

Cancer cells not only *look* different, they *are* different. Very different. An ordinary cell must acquire multiple capabilities to become a cancerous cell, and the last capability—to metastasize, or send pioneer cancer cells out to form new colonies at distant sites—is the deadliest, accounting for 90 percent of cancer deaths.[1] The concept of metastasis is a very important one. Without it, cancer probably won't kill you. With it, it very well might. Many treatments for cancer, especially complex cancers, are designed to contain the cancer and slow its progress. Doctor Armando Sardi, Doctor Paul Sugarbaker, and many of their colleagues have a different ambition: for a subset of cancers, if circumstances are favorable, they would like to *cure* the cancer, eliminate it completely and forever. Practically speaking, you almost can never be certain that cancer is gone, and gone for good, but setting *cure* as an ideal also happens to give the patient the best chance of survival in select cases.

Doctor Roenneburg's recommendation proved especially prescient, as Doctor Sardi is both a skilled surgeon and a skilled diagnostician. For example, by 2003 Carole Langrall, owner of the floral design business *A Garden of Earthly Delights,* the name inspired by the famous Hieronymus Bosch painting, had had her work displayed in numerous venues, including the American Visionary Art Museum and the Baltimore Museum of Art. She taught classes and had an active social life.

Carole experienced a series of symptoms, which her doctor began to treat with the standard protocol: beta blockers and a diuretic for her hypertension, and Topamax, an antiseizure medication, for her migraines. None of it worked. Over the next five years, she also experienced neuropathy, a loss of sensation in her hands and feet, memory lapses, mental fogginess, and extreme lethargy.

The nadir occurred when a gynecologist told her she was exaggerating her symptoms. Carole felt compelled to distance herself from family and friends who couldn't accept her illness.

Inspired by a doctor on *The Oprah Winfrey Show* who said that the body never lies, Carole asked her own doctor for a referral to see a cardiologist, Doctor Miriam Cohen of Baltimore, who treated her symptoms seriously. After a battery of tests, Cohen found that Carole's potassium levels were very low and that there was a nodule on one of her two adrenal glands.

Carole then recalled Doctor Sardi. Dan Collins, a member of Mercy Hospital's public relations staff and a freelance writer, previously had arranged for Carole to meet Sardi, to help him improve his English. Both Carole and Sardi had busy schedules, so the project didn't get far, but Sardi had made a good impression on her, telling her to let him know if she ever needed anything. She called him to receive a recommendation for a reliable endocrinologist.

Doctor Sardi gave her some names, but first read her medical history. He thought everything pointed to a rare adrenal condition called Conn's disease, which is marked by low levels of potassium, high blood pressure, and an overproduction of aldosterone, a hormone that balances the body's sodium and potassium levels. When these electrolytes are imbalanced, muscle coordination, the ability to concentrate, and heart and nerve function can get out of whack.

Doctor Sardi told Carole that removing the faulty adrenal gland probably would cure her, and that she probably would not need medication. She was apprehensive about facing surgery, but Sardi also happened to be a practitioner of laparoscopic, or minimally invasive, surgery. After he removed the affected adrenal gland, Carole's mental fogginess disappeared immediately, and she was released from the hospital after two days. She also went off six prescriptions.[2]

Lisa awoke from minor surgery for the second time.

She had been through a lot so far. First she had undergone a physical exam by Doctor Sardi, a man with a gentle demeanor and soft gray eyes. He spoke quietly to his associates, retaining the Spanish pronunciation of certain letters even when speaking English. Sometimes his speech also sped up considerably, reflecting a nuanced train of thought but making him even more difficult to understand. He was easiest to follow when he slowed down his speech and used his hands for emphasis, but even then, for many patients, medical terminology could be confounding.

Lisa's exam had taken place on a Friday. She then saw her primary care physician to receive a complete blood count test (CBC), a comprehensive metabolic panel blood test (CMP), an electrocardiogram (EKG), and a chest X-ray, with the results faxed to Mercy. The first blood test determined whether the blood counts were normal, and the second comprised fourteen standardized tests, including one to determine whether kidney and liver function were normal. The EKG measured the health of the heart. Lisa's heart, kidney, and liver functions had to be good for her to withstand prolonged surgery.

She then underwent a laparoscopic exam with Doctor Sardi. Laparoscopic surgery, sometimes called keyhole surgery, begins with a small incision in the abdomen. The abdominal cavity is then inflated, and a cold light source, usually halogen or xenon, is used for illumination. This surgery ensures less pain for the patient, promotes a faster recovery time, and has obvious cosmetic benefits.

When Lisa had awakened from that first surgery, Doctor Sardi told her he had found stage IV carcinomatosis throughout her abdominal cavity. Cancer was everywhere.

Worse, she also had cirrhosis of the liver. The cirrhosis in and of itself was not necessarily going to be a problem, but if the portal vein that ran through the liver were damaged, her liver probably would not withstand the trauma of a prolonged surgery. In medical parlance, she would not be a good candidate for surgery.

Mercy Hospital's chief of gastroenterology, Doctor Paul Thuluvath, would have to sign off on the liver; Doctor Sardi had arranged for it even before Lisa had awakened.

Not all patients who have peritoneal carcinomatosis and other cancers that often can be treated with cytoreductive surgery and hot chemo, such as appendiceal cancer, ovarian cancer, and colorectal cancer, are good candidates for surgery. The surgery is invasive, to say the least, and long, often ten hours or more. A patient must have the requisite organ function, the stamina, and the emotional strength to withstand the procedure. As Lisa was then age fifty-seven, she had a good chance of being a candidate.

The time leading up to her liver biopsy was fraught with anxiety. On the morning of that minor surgery, she poured out her heart to the attending nurse, much as she had done with Marcy when she had first learned about the cancer. With considerable compassion the nurse listened to everything Lisa had to say, which often proved to be the case at Mercy Hospital.

Doctor Thuluvath may have been told about her anxiety, as he was right there when Lisa awoke from minor surgery for the second time. "Everything's fine," he said. "I've already sent a text to Doctor Sardi to go ahead [with the major surgery]." Lisa was relieved and grateful; she would have a second chance at life after all.

The diagnosis, or identification, of cancer goes at least as far back as the age of Pericles, twenty-four centuries ago, when the Greek physician Hippocrates, noting the crablike appearance of a tumor, called cancer *karkinoma*, and its variant spelling, *carcinoma*, is still used today.[3] The word *cancer*, used by the first-century encyclopedist Aulus Cornelius Celsus, is the Roman translation of *crab*, and the words *oncology* and *oncologist*, used by the second century Greek physician Galen of Pergamon, comes from the Greek for *swelling*.

What was probably a case of breast cancer was also described in *The Edwin Smith Papyrus*, which dates back at least thirty-seven centuries, and this papyrus almost surely was copied from a now-lost document that was itself even older. Most of the document describes treatment for gaping wounds and head injuries, probably related to war, but case forty-five describes the bulging tumors on a male chest, likening the hardness and consistency to that of a green hemat fruit. It was the only malady in the manuscript for which there was no treatment.[4]

Thirteenth-century rabbi and physician Mosheh ben Maimon, whose writings also extended into the fields of law and ethics, described the process of removing a tumor and surrounding tissue but noted this was not possible in some cases: if the tumor contained a large blood supply, or if the tumor were too near a major organ.[5] In the eighteenth century, the famous Scottish surgeon John Hunter reiterated this assertion.

Until the late-nineteenth century, cutting out a tumor or trying to excise it with a heated piece of metal were the only treatments for cancer, in those instances when it was treated at all, but as the aforementioned Celsus noted, "After excision, even when a scar has formed, nonetheless the disease has returned, and caused death; while...the majority of patients, although no violent measures are applied in the attempt to remove the tumor, but only mild applications in order to soothe it, attain a ripe old age in spite of it."[6]

Over the centuries, doctors familiar with Celsus's observation often left cancer alone. For starters, until antiseptic was understood and widely used in the nineteenth century, any surgery carried the risk of death by infection. But this did not mean that cancer, or more precisely, the metastasis, or spreading of cancer, would kill the patient. Patients simply would die from something else before the cancer could run its course. Around 1900 or so, cancer was the seventh-leading cause of death in the United States. After World War II, after the conquest of so many diseases by the use of antibiotics, vaccines, and other methods, the

would deliberate further. Sardi told her he thought her odds of survival were 80 percent.

Both videos end with a brief mention of the annual September reunion of Doctor Sardi's former patients, which begins with a reception and silent auction on the first floor of Mercy Hospital's Weinberg Center on a Saturday, followed by a fundraising walk, *Heat It to Beat It*, around the Baltimore Inner Harbor on the subsequent Sunday.

What is likely to capture the popular imagination more than anything else is the hot chemo bath. But of the important factors involved in these successful cases, the chemo bath is only one of five: the accuracy of the diagnosis, the skill of the surgeon and the center, the completeness of the cytoreductive surgery, the chemo bath, and the subsequent chemotherapy follow-up. Although Doctor Sardi at one point called the hot chemo bath the most important factor, not all oncologists, even among advocates for HIPEC, necessarily agree with that.[12]

It may seem a bit odd that so many sources cite the hot chemo bath, or HIPEC, as being "controversial," "experimental," or both. When, in 1767, the famed surgeon John Hunter injected himself with gonorrhea and wound up with both gonorrhea and syphilis, it was experimental. When, in 1924, Russian physician and science-fiction writer Alexander Bogdanov took eleven infusions of blood to arrest his balding and improve his eyesight, but instead contracted malaria and tuberculosis, it was experimental. The same term may seem out of place for a procedure that has now been performed many thousands of times and is currently offered in more than two hundred centers worldwide.

In a series of interviews, Doctor Sardi rejected the notion that the hot chemo bath is experimental. "Some insurance company called it experimental treatment," he said, "which is not true." When asked if chemotherapy is considered the standard treatment, he replied, "For peritoneal carcinomatosis many people think so, although the results with chemotherapy alone are very poor...They are much better with cytoreductive surgery, HIPEC, and intravenous chemotherapy afterward."[13]

One reason for the "experimental" label is that the track record for HIPEC varies according to the type of cancer being treated. At Mercy Hospital, Doctor Sardi and his colleague, Doctor Vadim Gushchin, use HIPEC to treat patients with peritoneal carcinomatosis of the colon, rectum, stomach, appendix, and ovaries, as well as mesotheliomas, sarcomas, and primary peritoneal cancers. The success rate varies not only with the origin of the cancer but also with the staging (I-IV), indexing, and lymph node metastasis.

One possible reason that the acceptance of HIPEC has been slow is that it has gone by at least twelve different names.[14] At the Fourth International Workshop on Peritoneal Surface Malignancy held in Madrid in 2004, an attempt was made to get the alphabet soup down to a single acronym, HIPEC, which met with mixed success.

Another reason HIPEC is considered experimental is because there are so many variations in its administration. The bath itself can last thirty to 120 minutes; the temperature used can vary as much as 3° centigrade[15]; the bath can be delivered in many ways; and even the specific drugs used can vary. Further, the concentrations of chemotherapy used could be *twenty to one thousand times*[16] greater than intravenous chemo, as very little of the large molecule doses would be absorbed through the peritoneum and into the bloodstream, ensuring less cytotoxicity. Until very recently, and to a certain extent even now, medical procedures were not supposed to be like hairdressing or fashion design. Uniformity was sought. There was, and is, a constant struggle to define standard care and to get regulatory bodies and insurance companies to sign off on it.

More important, achieving standard-care status means demonstrating that HIPEC works better than alternative treatments, or when there are no alternative treatments, that it works better than no treatment at all. Standard care is ascertained through the use of clinical trials and randomized, controlled studies. The clinical trial uses the scientific method and compares two groups or more, isolating one key factor. An early, notable clinical trial was conducted by James Lind, a Scottish surgeon in the Royal Navy who sought a cure for scurvy.[17]

Scurvy, a disease that in its final stages can cause tooth loss, loss of sensation in the hands and feet, pus-filled wounds, fever and death, was long ago identified by Hippocrates and became very common among sailors and pirates during the Age of Discovery, which required longer times at sea.

Lind, who later would initiate preventative measures for typhus and would discover that distilled salt water was suitable for drinking, divided twelve men who showed initial signs of scurvy into six groups of two. All had the same diet, but the first group was given a quart of cider every day; the second, twenty-five drops of oil of vitriol; the third, six spoonfuls of vinegar; the fourth, half a pint of seawater; the fifth, two oranges and one lemon; and the sixth, spicy paste with barley water. After six days, with the citrus fruit used up, one of the men in group five was cured, and the other had recovered significantly. Within the rules, regulations, and safeguards of today's medical practice, this experiment would not now qualify as a medical trial, but it's still useful for illustrative purposes.

And it eventually saved lives.

For the most part, the protocol of today's randomized clinical trials goes back about sixty-five years. One enormously influential work was *Effectiveness & Efficiency: Random Reflections on Health Services*, published in 1972 by Scottish epidemiologist Archie Cochrane. Since 1993 the Cochrane Collaboration, with more than 28,000 volunteers in one hundred countries, has sought to organize medical research in a systematic way.

Cochrane's own experience, first with an ambulance unit in the Spanish Civil War and later as a medical officer during World War II, convinced him that nothing being offered to tuberculosis patients helped them, and some remedies were perhaps counterproductive. He wanted to use the scientific method in the clinical trial to change that.

In fact the first randomized clinical trial did prove effective against tuberculosis, though that 1948 trial was conducted by epidemiologist Sir Austin Bradford Hill, who had been influenced by Ronald Almer Fisher's agricultural experiments using the same methodology. In Hill's trial, half the tuberculosis patients were treated with streptomycin, which proved to be the first antibiotic to be effective in treating TB.[18]

A decade or so after Cochrane penned his work, Doctor David M. Eddy used clinical trials to investigate whether procedures then in use were effective. He found that many of them, including the conventional treatments for back pain and glaucoma, bone-marrow transplants for breast cancer, and many forms of heart surgery, simply didn't work.[19]

There are considerable safeguards to clinical trials. Patients must give their informed consent, which primarily means that the possible risks and benefits have been explained to them.[20] A patient may drop out of a clinical trial at any time, though this may be inadvisable, especially if he or she is experiencing adverse side effects. Patients must first be offered established treatment, if available, in conjunction with the trial procedure. And if one of the treatments or procedures proves clearly superior, or inferior, during a trial, the trial will be shut down early, and all participants may opt for the better treatment. There is a great deal of oversight, especially in Europe, Japan, and the United States.[21]

Nonetheless, nearly one-third of all clinical trials fail to attract a single participant. And in the critical Phase III trials, it's possible that up to 60 percent do not attract enough applicants to be completed.[22]

All these layers of patient protection, in addition to the difficulty of finding enough patients to finish, or even begin, a study, means that many clinical trials are done in countries with significantly less oversight. It is sad that the safeguards afforded to citizens of the United States and most developed countries are not always granted overseas, a controversial topic.[23]

For most patients faced with difficult decisions regarding their own care, understanding a little about Phase II and Phase III clinical trials should suffice, though there are Phase Ø, Phase I, Phase 1b, and Phase IV trials as well.[24]

In Phase II studies, the new drugs or procedures already have been tested on animals, and safe dosages have been determined for patients. The next question to be answered is whether the new treatment is better than the standard treatment, if there is one, and often a relatively small number of patients are treated. Some Phase II studies are randomized, but most are not.

In Phase III studies, the new drugs or procedures are compared to the current standard treatment in a rigorous randomized study. Patients who sign up for a Phase III trial are informed about the two, occasionally more, options, called "arms," of the study that are available to them. They will know about the survival rates and side effects that emerged from the Phase II studies. What they will not know, and when feasible, what their doctors will not know, is in which arm of the study they will be. The patient must be about equally comfortable with each of the options available.

Whereas the randomized, controlled trial, in theory legitimately offers the highest standard of proof, in practice it is often difficult to find patients who are equally comfortable with both options, and as a result, the current data regarding the effectiveness of HIPEC in randomized trials was apparently limited to three published studies as of 2011, at the point where Lisa had to make her decision. In one study of sixty-eight colorectal cancer patients in Japan, half were given HIPEC. The patients in this group lived an average of fourteen days longer than the control group, statistically significant, but small comfort to patients weighing the HIPEC option.

The other two studies are a little more convincing. Between March 1987 and December 1996, at a time when the administration of HIPEC wasn't as sophisticated as it is today, 141 gastric carcinoma patients in Japan were split into two groups, those who received surgery and those who received both surgery and intraperitoneal hyperthermic chemoperfusion (IHCP), which would now be considered HIPEC. The survival rate was 10 percent better in the IHCP group.[25] In a very small study in the Netherlands for colorectal cancer patients, progression-free survival was 39 percent longer and disease-specific survival 75 percent longer for the CTR + HIPEC group than the control group.[26]

Though the requisite proof is admittedly thin, there are many abstracts indicating the effectiveness of HIPEC that are outside the strict parameters of a clinical trial. One major study of appendix cancer has suggested that cytoreductive surgery and HIPEC should be considered standard practice. Another paper out of Australia suggested that cytoreductive surgery and HIPEC should be considered the standard of care in many cases of colorectal cancer. In the Netherlands HIPEC has been the standard of care for PMP, appendiceal cancer, since 1995.[27]

There was a randomized, controlled study open in the United States with the National Institutes of Health (NIH) for more than two years, but although the study was designed for more than three hundred patients, only one signed up. One. The reason should not be hard to guess; most people who take a look at the results of HIPEC decline to participate in such a study, as no one wants to be in the randomized group that *doesn't* receive the HIPEC.

Doctor Jesus Esquivel of Saint Agnes Hospital is a colleague of Doctor Armando Sardi as well as of Doctor Paul Sugarbaker of the Washington Cancer Center; Dr. Sugarbaker is a pioneer in several types of cancer treatment. In his presentations Esquivel used to use the following humorous analogy to illustrate the dilemma.

Parachute use to prevent death and major trauma related to gravitational challenge: systematic review of randomised controlled trials[28]

The aforementioned title appeared in the *British Medical Journal* in December 2003. Is the use of a parachute really beneficial to people who jump from airplanes? A simplification: the study divides potential volunteers into two equal groups, those who jump from an airplane with a parachute and those who do not. All volunteers must be about equally comfortable with either option. No one volunteers for the study, which does not deter the formulation of a conclusion:

Parachutes appear to reduce the risk of injury after gravitational challenge, but their effectiveness has not been proven.

Doctor Paul H. Sugarbaker, author of more than 850 published articles and a host of textbooks, one of which, *Peritoneal Carcinomatosis: Principles of Management*, has been translated into five languages, has cast his shadow not only upon cytoreductive surgery but also upon every HIPEC procedure performed in the world today. In fact the use of cytoreductive surgery with HIPEC is still sometimes referred to as the "Sugarbaker protocol" or even the "Sugarbaker procedure,"[29] but history has not always practiced the fidelity it could. Sports surgeon Frank Jobe, for example, introduced elbow ligament reconstruction, but the surgery is now called Tommy John surgery, named after a baseball pitcher who lay inert upon the operating table. Even so, a November 12, 2012 slide show put together by the *Washington Post* revived, or possibly even introduced, the term "Sugarbaker procedure" in the United States.

Doctor Sugarbaker is not as circuitous as Doctor Esquivel. In speaking of peritoneal mesothelioma, he said, "There are no randomized controlled studies, and there never will be. And if the medical oncologists keep asking for evidence-based medicine, they're not going to get it."[30]

Doctor Sardi is equally adamant. More than 80 percent of the patients who come to see him already have had one or more failed therapies and sometimes multiple failed surgeries as well. These antecedents not only make it more difficult for Sardi and his team to be successful but also increase the chances for complications. "How are you going to tell someone that there is a 50 percent chance that they will get something that has already failed and also that they will *not* get something that works?"

Author Devra Davis succinctly describes the problem of practical necessity trumping consensual proof.

When a patient shows up with a bad headache, a physician cannot say come back in five years when I've completed my research and we'll figure out what to do. Many medical problems are inherently emergent—they require answers on the spot. Regarding how best to find cancer and what treatments make sense to try, the use of scientific information to evaluate what works is more limited than most of us realize.[31]

Not everyone who consults with Doctor Sardi receives a recommendation of HIPEC. "We have moved from very radical surgeries to more confined surgeries," he explains. "Not everyone has the same tumor, the same size, the same location. Some people talk about radical surgeries as something bad, but ...we [only] use radical surgery for people who need it."

However, for many of the patients who come to him, Doctor Sardi is convinced that HIPEC is the only real choice. "The majority of patients that come to us come very late," he says. "They come after many surgeries, after multiple rounds of chemotherapy, and most are markedly debilitated. This is a big operation, and people can die from this operation. We only had one mortality, from a seventy-six-year-old woman who suffered a heart attack in 1998. Complications do occur, but we can handle them most of the time without problems. Not everyone is going to be cured either. The treatment has the possibility of having severe complications, as you can imagine, but the alternative is death, so it's not like we have a good choice and a not so good choice— we have a *terrible* choice or one that is pretty good but has some risk to get there.

"Really this is an extensive operation. There are multiple procedures taking place. It takes twelve, fourteen hours of actual surgery. It requires several days of recovery, and most of these patients feel that we run a truck over them, and in fact we do. It takes two months for them to go back to normal, but we are here to support them."

Two

*At every step you take it will feel as if you are treading upon
sharp knives, and that the blood must flow. If you will bear all
this, I will help you. --from Hans Christian Andersen's The
Little Mermaid*

Doctor Paul Sugarbaker was born in Baltimore in 1941
but went to grade school in Jefferson City, Missouri. He
earned his Bachelor of Science degree in chemistry at Wheaton
College, Illinois, about twenty-five miles west of the heart of
Chicago. He graduated from medical school at Cornell and later
received his master's degree in immunology from Harvard. In
1999 he received an honorary doctorate from l'Université de
Liège in the French community of Liège, Belgium.

One professional website, http://www.omicsonline.org, contains the following description of him. "Doctor Sugarbaker is a
strong critic of current surgical tradition. He believes that major
changes in the technology of cancer resection are necessary...
His theme, 'It's what the surgeon doesn't see that kills the patient,' summarizes the concepts behind his 850 publications in

the oncology literature." Sugarbaker knows that a percentage of all cancers in the abdominal and pelvic area will have metastasized elsewhere in the peritoneum and that the oncologist who doesn't address this is doing the patient a major disservice.

Fifteen years ago, even ten years ago, it would not have been unfair to characterize Doctor Sugarbaker as a maverick intellectual heavyweight haunting the primeval ivory towers of American medical orthodoxy. In 2013 it probably would be more accurate to refer to him as a mainstream intellectual heavyweight welcomed in the conference rooms of many modern American treatment centers. He was just a little ahead of his time. Even if the term "the Sugarbaker procedure" never completely catches on, a century or more from now, students of surgery may well know him as the father of cytoreductive surgery.

It is part of his nature to be ahead of the curve. Early in his career, one of his mentors was Doctor Joseph Murray, who would go on to share a Nobel Prize in Medicine or Physiology with Doctor E. Donnall Thomas in 1990. In 1954 Murray performed the first successful kidney transplant. Murray's real passion, however, was plastic surgery, and he reconstructed many of the hands and faces of World War II veterans.

Doctor Murray made a big impression on the younger Sugarbaker when he told him that the way to be successful at surgical problem solving was to become an expert in a well-defined field, to help develop the field, and to ask in-depth questions. Sugarbaker began to cast about for something that was cutting edge.

Doctor Sugarbaker was an intern and later a resident at Peter Bent Brigham Hospital shortly after Michael Gold and Samuel O. Freeman published their work on CEA, a glycoprotein, which, at elevated levels, could indicate the presence of cancer, what oncologists call a tumor marker. Sugarbaker became the CEA blood-test coordinator, walking about the hospital with blood samples in his pocket and asking the big questions: What was the role of CEA in determining prognosis? What was the role in the diagnosis of recurrence in follow-up? And so on. The manuscripts he helped put together to demonstrate the role that CEA should play in colorectal cancer management proved successful. His group could predict the recurrence of cancer about six months before it would show up on a CT scan.

Doctor Sugarbaker then had a chance for a brief fellowship in New York with the Japanese-born Doctor Hiromi Shinya. Shinya was then pioneering colonoscopic techniques, a field that was in its infancy. In fact Shinya began doing colonoscopies with an esophagoscope until the Olympus Optical Company introduced a dedicated colonoscope in 1969. Shinya felt polyps were often a precursor to cancer, and because he wanted to remove them with noninvasive surgery, he collaborated with Olympus engineer Hiroshi Ichikawa to invent a surgical snare,[1] still in use today, which brought him worldwide fame in the medical world.

For years Sugarbaker was apparently the only doctor in New England who even had a colonoscope. He made movies so medical personnel anywhere in the world could learn how to perform a colonoscopy and how to remove polyps. Favorable articles in peer-reviewed journals helped spread the word.[2]

As they say in show biz, he had arrived.

Doctor Sugarbaker had the chance to do more surgical problem solving at the National Institutes of Health in Bethesda, Maryland, first as a senior investigator and later as the head of the colorectal cancer section. Colorectal cancer is one of the most stubborn of the cancers that can be found in the peritoneum. It resists chemo. It recurs. By the time it reaches stage IV, sometimes referred to as "signet ring" because of the appearance of the cancer cells, there's significantly less hope for the patient. The genesis of what would become cytoreductive surgery was surely formulated during those years. He was also ahead of the curve in the treatment of colorectal cancer that had spread to the liver, a surgery few surgeons would go anywhere near, either because they were concerned about too much bleeding or because they assumed, often wrongly, that any cancer that had spread to the liver also must have spread systemically, or just about everywhere in the body.

In 1996 Doctor Sugarbaker published *Peritoneal Carcinomatosis: Principals and Management*, the textbook that has been translated into five languages. The synopsis notes that except in a few patients with ovarian cancer, which is more responsive to drugs than other abdominal cancers, peritoneal carcinomatosis, the very diagnosis Lisa would receive years later, was a terminal condition. Sugarbaker suggested that with aggressive management, new techniques, and new technology, a complete eradication of the disease could occur.

His own observations confirmed what encyclopedist Aulus Cornelius Celsus had noted almost two millennia previously—that after the surgical removal of a tumor, the tumor returns anyway, even "if a scar has formed." Coupled with Paget's observations after the autopsies of 735 women who had died of breast cancer—that the metastasis of the disease can be found in the same old, reliable places,[3] Sugarbaker apparently decided to pursue the concept that the metastasis of abdominal cancer was also as predictable.

In investigating twenty-one sarcoma patients who had supposedly had their primary tumors completely removed, but for whom cancer had returned, he made several observations. One type of cancer cell was always found along the incision lines. The trauma of surgery causes the proliferation of fibrin along these lines, normally a good thing in terms of the healing process. But cancer cells could embed themselves in this fibrin and, thus protected, would be insensitive to future chemotherapy treatments.

Doctor Sugarbaker's observation on this matter was not without precedent. As far back as the 1860s, London's Doctor Charles Moore charted the recurrence of cancer for breast cancer patients. There, too, cancer had recurred near the incision lines. Unfortunately Moore came to the wrong conclusion—that the entire breast and sometimes even the surrounding areas needed to be completely removed.[4] Surgery alone—or for that matter, radiation alone—simply cannot solve the problem of metastasis.

Doctor Sugarbaker also broke down the abdominal cavity into nine abdominopelvic regions, and twenty-one sites were scored for a second type of cancer, which looked different from the cancer that had formed along the incision lines. In the first surgery, this second type of cancer had been found in an average of 1.81 of the nine regions. Now he was finding it in an average of 5.13 of the nine regions.

When cancer cells disengage from the primary tumor, they seek out two things in their future colonies—a place with room to grow continuously, at least for awhile, and a place where they also can get the blood supply necessary for their survival. Sugarbaker catalogued these same old, reliable places, one of the most notable of which is the peritoneal surface itself, a membrane that encases the lower half of the torso.[5]

In January 2000, biologists Douglas Hanahan and Robert A. Weinberg published a watershed work, "The Hallmarks of Cancer." Prior to its publication, the previous twenty-five years of cancer research had been bewildering; the authors use the term "complex almost beyond measure."[6] Building upon the earlier work of British biologist Leslie Foulds, who in 1954 noted that tumorigenesis, the progression of normal cells to cancerous cells, is a multistage process,[7] Hanahan and Weinberg stated that there are six capabilities necessary for rogue cells to become cancerous, and each of these six capabilities manages to bypass the body's natural anticancer defenses.

Almost all cells in the human body have a bit more than thirty thousand genes. Some of these genes have been identified as oncogenes; when abnormally activated, they can cause cancer. Still, there are six things that must happen for a cell to become cancerous. Though the analogy is a simplification, if someone needed six different passwords to access your computer, they might never get in.

First, normal cells await growth signals to replicate. These growth signals help ensure that a given type of cell will replicate as often as needed, no more and no less. But oncogenes within a cell can mimic this growth signal, disrupting the proper behavior of the cell. There are actually several strategies for accomplishing this, the most insidious being to induce normal neighboring cells to release growth-stimulating signals. No longer needing to await "permission" to replicate, the cell can divide freely and continually.

Second, normal cells are sensitive to *antigrowth* signals, and there are several of these signals that the cell needs to bypass to become cancerous.

Third, normal cells are programmed for apoptosis, or cell death. A number of things can trigger apoptosis, including DNA damage and inadequate oxygen supply. A shorthand way of looking at this is that cells wear out: white blood cells wear out quickly; bone cells wear out very slowly. Drifting away from a cell's designated area also causes apoptosis in most cells, ensuring "architectural" integrity throughout the body. Just as a cell can avoid growth signals, a cell can avoid death by using a different variety of strategies. For example, in many colon cancer and lung cancer cell lines, which are especially resilient, the strategy involves uploading decoy receptors so the cell never gets the "message" that it's time to die.

At this point it would seem that the conditions for cancer growth are sufficient. The cell can replicate without restrictions, evade signals to stop replicating, and evade signals that it's time to die. The fourth obstacle, however, is that even when external signals for growth can be ignored, most and perhaps all cells have a backup autonomous program for growth; this mechanism must also be evaded. With each division, telomeres at the end of each chromosome get a little shorter. As with the wick of a candle that can burn for only so long, normal cells can replicate themselves only sixty to seventy times, which is sometimes referred to as the Hayflick limit.[8] Cancerous cells produce an enzyme called telomerase that rebuilds telomeres. Cancerous cells can have no limitations. They can be immortal.

The fifth obstacle to be breached has to do with the fact that blood washes past every cell in the body, delivering oxygen and nutrients and carrying away refuse. As cells are dependent on nearby capillaries, the smallest of the blood vessels, intuition might suggest that normal cells would have angiogenic ability, the ability to encourage nearby blood-vessel growth. But they don't. Cancerous cells do. Unlike normal cells, they can spread to parts unknown, but mostly to the same old predictable, reliable places, creating their own blood supply as they replicate. Here, too, the strategies vary in "turning on the angiogenic switch," and complicating things, the strategies seem to vary in different kinds of cancers.

The sixth and last obstacle cells must overcome is the issue of metastasis, or sending pioneer cancer cells out to form new colonies at distant sites. As mentioned in the previous chapter, this last factor accounts for 90 percent of cancer deaths. The adherence mechanism to adjacent tissue must be disabled. This can happen in multiple ways, depending on the tissue. There is more to this sixth capability than merely the cancerous cells' ability to "break free," but these other capabilities are perhaps the least understood of the six conditions for normal cells to become invasive.

It may seem counterintuitive that cancer cells, which can bring death, can be immortal, but normal cells are not. The 1912 Nobel Prize–winning biologist, surgeon, and eugenicist Alexis Carrel claimed to have kept a chicken heart alive for more than twenty years. His theory was that *all* cells can replicate themselves forever if the right environment or culture can be found. Renowned anatomist Leonard Hayflick later disproved his theory, and no one since has been able to reproduce his chicken-heart experiment. But it did turn out that cells *could* become immortal, or replicate themselves without restriction, if abnormally changed. The first cell line that proved immortal was cultured by a Johns Hopkins scientist named George Gey and was taken from a woman dying of cervical cancer, Henrietta Lacks, a story captured by Rebecca Skloot in the nonfiction book *The Immortal Life of Henrietta Lacks.* The cervical cancer cells taken from Henrietta Lacks, referred to as HeLa cells or hela cells, have been replicating rapidly and continually since 1951. One scientist has estimated that there are now more than fifty million metric tons in one place or another. HeLa cells have been used extensively in research, from the testing of the polio vaccine to research in cancer, AIDS and the effects of radiation, to name just a few. HeLa cells have also been used in gene mapping and in defining cancer markers.[9]

Many of the future strategies in fighting cancer will include *earlier* diagnosis, more *accurate* diagnosis, *less expensive* diagnosis, and *earlier* treatment. Some of this is happening now, albeit incrementally. For Doctor Sugarbaker in the 1980s and 1990s, there was a more immediate problem, one that probably never will be irrelevant, even with earlier interventions; how do you keep these cancers of the peritoneum from recurring?

Doctor Sugarbaker introduced of a pair of similar techniques—early postoperative intraperitoneal chemotherapy (EPIC) and intraperitoneal regional chemotherapy (IPRC), the forerunner of today's HIPEC. A precedent for those techniques had been established with successful experiments by Doctor John Spratt, professor of surgery at the University of Louisville, Kentucky, and reported in 1980. Spratt is probably best known in oncology circles as a successful breast cancer surgeon who participated in the debate regarding the usefulness of mammograms.[10]

Doctor Spratt worked out a system to treat spreading cancer within the thin membrane that surrounds the abdominal cavity by applying chemotherapy heated to 41° C (105.8° F) and safely applied his system to fifteen dogs. He then used the system on a thirty-five-year-old man after surgery for pseudomyxoma peritonei (PMP), a form of appendix cancer. This time the chemotherapy circulated at 42° C for ninety minutes. The procedure was repeated eight days later, and the man's recovery was reported to be uneventful, without major complications. Subsequently papers about the experiments with the dogs and the successful treatment of the man were published simultaneously.[11]

At the time Marie Muskovin was working as a cancer control nurse with Doctor Spratt under a grant with the National Institutes of Health. Her role during the course of the patient's surgery was to remind Spratt when to take samples and to make sure the samples were processed correctly. She was aware of the historic nature of the operation at the time and noted that Spratt was able to grow cancer cells from the distillate, or concentrated essence, of the surgery. She also noted that the patient recovered remarkably quickly and was alive and cancer free when she left the university four or five years later. It seems odd that after all that research Spratt only performed one surgery, but Muskovin said he wanted to be very, very selective. One possibility is that his patient was a professional colleague whose condition was otherwise terminal and, familiar with the experiments on canines, convinced Spratt to do the operation. Another possibility is that Spratt did those fifteen surgeries on dogs precisely to save a colleague's life.

From 1996 on, after Doctor Sugarbaker published his landmark book on the treatment of peritoneal carcinomatosis, the literature on HIPEC available in medical journals exploded. When I last checked in 2013, there were more than 500 abstracts in the literature; these abstracts can be accessed by scrolling down the resources tab at http://www.hipectreatment.com.

For Doctor Sugarbaker the most important pieces had fallen into place. It was not enough to remove the primary tumor if the cancer had metastasized. One had to thoroughly remove *all* tumor from the entire abdominal cavity; this included performing a peritonectomy, a massive operation in and of itself, which could include up to six procedures.[12] Such an operation could take anywhere from ten to fourteen hours. Though results would depend heavily on the amount of cancer present at the beginning of the surgery, in general if a surgeon could get it all, the patient's long-term prognosis was very good. If a surgeon could get almost all of it, months or years would be added to the patient's life.

For subsequent chemotherapy to work, the nodules remaining had to be very small, possibly two millimeters or shorter, or else the chemotherapy would not necessarily penetrate. To get these very small nodules, as well as the spilled cancer cells that otherwise would embed themselves along the incision lines, chemotherapy had to be applied right away. As mentioned, much higher concentrations, twenty to one thousand times as much, could be applied to the abdominal cavity immediately after surgery than could be applied intravenously later, and heating the solution could greatly enhance the potency of many, but not all, chemotherapy regimens.[13] The temperature selected, that of hot bathwater, was about the hottest that normal cells would tolerate. Even with this, while the chemo is maintained at 43° C, the body must be maintained at about 37° C to prevent fever. In theory, at least so far, this was the best chance yet at long-term survival for patients with many forms of peritoneal cancer.

European and Japanese oncologists took up the cudgels very early on; at one point Doctor Vadim Guchshin, Doctor Sardi's partner, quipped that the entire European medical community lived in Doctor Sugarbaker's basement. Yet it took quite a while for Sugarbaker's ideas to catch on in the United States. A best-selling work, *Everyone's Guide to Cancer Therapy*, fifth edition, which otherwise does a good job of explaining complex concepts to laypersons, as of 2013 makes no mention of cytoreductive surgery or HIPEC.

There always have been legitimate questions. How safe is HIPEC? For the patient, are the possible complications tolerable? Are the benefits worth the risk? And so on. With all that, sheer stubbornness may have been a factor in the slow recognition of Doctor Sugarbaker's work. One oncologist likened HIPEC to the SUV; when sport-utility vehicles first came out, companies such as Porsche and Mercedes made a point of *not* producing them, though they eventually relented, at least for awhile.

Something else: Doctor Sugarbaker was asking a great deal from the front-line doctors, many surgeons, and maybe even the patients themselves.

Many doctors either misdiagnose cancers of the peritoneum or tell patients there is no treatment. Even prestigious cancer centers have made mistakes. Laurie Todd, author of *Fight Your Health Insurer and Win*, a book designed to help people when a claim for complex surgery is denied by their insurance company,[14] writes:

> When my oncologist told me there was no treatment, and that I had two good years left, my first impulse was to do some research and find out if this was really true. It turned out not to be true. Since then, I have learned that not every patient reacts this way. Many would not conceive of questioning their doctor. They would accept the two years with grace, suffer and die on schedule.[15]

Later, when her slides were sent to Johns Hopkins Hospital, she was informed that what she had was benign and not cancer, though that probably wasn't a misdiagnosis of what the slides contained at the time.

Doctor Sugarbaker was asking a lot from surgeons too. The cutting involved required very precise surgical techniques, almost requiring the surgeons to have a second sense of where one tissue ends and another begins. These surgeries also required a good team, ensuring the requisite oxygen supply, blood supply, and anesthetic dose be correctly administered at all times.

The amount of stamina required to perform these extremely long operations was certainly a potential stumbling block. Doctor Sugarbaker would let no one else, not even an experienced surgeon, perform any part of the surgeries for which he was responsible. The fact that Sugarbaker, born in 1941, has maintained such an exhausting pace for as long as he has is remarkable.

More than anything else, no two cases are exactly alike. A surgeon can be as much as two hours into the surgery before the puzzle becomes completely clear. What *precisely* needs to be resected, or removed, what *precisely* needs to be restored, and how is the patient to be reassembled so as to enjoy the highest quality of life under the circumstances? Doctor Gushchin observed that it took him sixty or seventy surgeries before he became comfortable with the procedures. A recently published study indicates that it may take up to 140 operations for a surgeon to master the procedures, though a subsequent publication by members of the same group was less demanding.[16]

The surgeon must make very difficult decisions. Female patients may very well lose their reproductive function, though not all do,[17] and men and women both may lose enough of their intestines to necessitate a colostomy or an ileostomy, both of which require the patient to affix a bag to the abdomen to collect solid waste. Many surgeons would prefer to focus on palliative measures, lesser surgery that would alleviate the pain and perhaps add some time to the patient's life.

Patients may face conflicting advice. Author Laurie Todd was in that position in 2003. She received conflicting recommendations within her network, and going out of her network, she eventually got another opinion entirely. Todd writes:

One name cropped up everywhere I looked—Doctor Paul Sugarbaker. He had started thirty-five years ago as a colon cancer surgeon at NIH, then put together a unique surgery and chemotherapy approach, applying the heated chemotherapy agents directly to the organs during the operation. He had performed this surgery over nine hundred times over twenty-five years on patients with my type of disease [pseudomyxoma peritonei, a form of appendicitis cancer]. All of a sudden I felt like Chicken Little, running around asking if the sky were falling. These doctors with their ovarian cancer and their months to live and their no cancer and their 30 percent could not all be right. And yet, each one spoke as if he were absolutely sure.[18]

In 2007 one of Doctor Sugarbaker's patients, Randolph N., who is himself a doctor, was diagnosed with mucinous adenoma, a form of appendix cancer. In comparing the five-year survival rates of Sugarbaker's patients and Memorial Sloan-Kettering patients, he found an 80 percent survival rate for Sugarbaker's patients and a 10 percent survival rate at Memorial Sloan-Kettering, even though it was rated as one of the four most prestigious cancer centers in the country, making his decision regarding treatment of this particular cancer very easy. Like many others, Randolph N. was initially denied treatment by his insurance company, though his wife, Lori, won on appeal.

Lisa was wheeled into the operating room.

She had been at the hospital for almost twenty-four hours, having arrived early on a Monday morning. Almost a month prior to her arrival, Doctor Sardi's then HIPEC coordinator, Jennifer Francis, had taken care of all of Lisa's insurance paperwork and had given her a book, *Carcinomatosis/HIPEC: Patient Resource Guide*, so she would have a better idea of what to expect.

The guide, which can be downloaded from the Mercy Hospital website, does an excellent job of getting the patient physically ready for therapy, and letting the patient know exactly what he or she will need. Lisa and I had put off one of the recommendations, bringing a bathrobe, until the day before she reported for care. I could have, and in retrospect should have, gotten one for her, but for some reason I thought she would enjoy picking out something she really liked for herself.

I parked as close to the store as I could, but the walk there proved laborious, necessitating many stops. She told me later she should have been in a wheelchair. None of the bathrobes in the women's section fit, and after putting on a heavy, navy-blue man's bathrobe, she broke down in tears.

It was everything. The excruciating walk to get there. The one month of going to work in pain, telling her coworkers everything would turn out fine, and hoping that saying so aloud would help make it come true. The immanence of the surgery. The embarrassment of having to wear a man's bathrobe. The startled clerk, a young lady, was confused, and it wasn't easy for me to explain to her that it was not anything she had done wrong.

On the fifteenth floor, Lisa's nurse had shown her how everything worked, and as the day wore on, several specialists came in to talk to her. Doctor Sardi stopped in with an assistant, Doctor Suven Shankar, to talk about the possibility of DNA profiling[19] and to ask her to donate the remnants of the surgery for research.

Visitors included Lisa's sole sibling, Steve, and his wife, Jacquie, who had traveled to be on hand, as well as a colleague, Doug, who brought some Mylar balloons to bring a bit of cheeriness to the room. Lisa was raised to show good manners under such circumstances. The conversation was light, carefree. She was merely being a good sport, as she was terrified.

In the evening, Lisa drank some god-awful stuff to cleanse her colon. Several times during the process, she was certain she could swallow not a single drop more, not one, and implored her nurse to come up with something else, anything else, but to no avail. This would prove to be a recurring motif; nurses and staff would listen with the utmost patience to suggested changes to the various protocols, but the protocols would remain unaltered.

In Hans Christian Andersen's fairy tale "The Little Mermaid," the youngest mermaid allows the sea witch to cut out her tongue; in the process the mermaid loses her voice. Each step she takes thereafter brings sharp pain. She makes such a bargain for a chance at a prince's hand in marriage and for an immortal soul. If he were to marry another, she would forfeit kindred, home, and the three hundred years afforded the life of a mermaid and instead become the white frothy foam upon the sea. Hers is a courageous decision, and although she does not win the prince's hand, her courage is nonetheless rewarded.

For a patient in Lisa's shoes, a courageous decision is also required. The surgery before her was not without danger; the recovery was sure to be long and trying; she might well have to learn how to live with a reorganized body; and with all that, the procedure was not guaranteed to work.

A few cancers have been cured, but by and large the cancer survivor lives in a shadow, for metastatic cancer usually recurs, even after several years. Valerie M., age forty-five in 2007, became too fatigued to work the dinner shift at one of her two restaurants in a small town in New York State. Previously she had worked around the clock. A concerned customer made her an appointment to see Doctor Elizabeth Gregory in nearby Stone

Ridge. After taking a CT scan, Gregory was candid; Valerie had ovarian cancer. She needed to get her affairs in order. Gregory also informed her about a $1,100-per-month life insurance policy for people who had preexisting conditions.

In Albany surgeons removed two melon-size tumors, but there was more bad news; the surgeons had discovered stage IV appendiceal cancer.

An Internet search by Valerie's brother Tom led to Doctor Armando Sardi. She visited him in Baltimore and was informed of cytoreductive surgery and HIPEC. Sardi told her she had a twenty percent chance of surviving. She noted that one of Sardi's very first cytoreductive surgery patients was still alive and felt confident in him. She also shored up her own confidence by saying that *somebody* had to be in that twenty percent. She went home for several months of chemotherapy then returned to Baltimore in March 2008 for an eleven-hour surgery. She and her sister Melissa stayed for three weeks near Mercy Hospital in the American Cancer Society Hope Lodge, a facility that has twenty-six rooms and serves all Baltimore-area hospitals. Within two years Valerie was back to working around the clock.

The extra years of life changed her perspective. In addition to managing her restaurants, she donated to charities, helped with school fundraisers, and acted as a mentor to newly diagnosed cancer patients. In spite of her courageous efforts, Valerie succumbed to the cancer in March 2012, five years after her initial diagnosis, and was buried near her home in Saint Mary of the Snow Cemetery.

Lisa had vague memories of the time when she was about ten and her mother was away from home off and on. Her grandmother and aunt busied themselves in the house, and Lisa wondered what was happening to her mother. Years later she found out that her mother had been treated for breast cancer, had undergone a double mastectomy and multiple rounds of chemotherapy, and had gone on to survive another thirty years. Lisa and I were planning a seventy-fifth birthday party for her mother when she died.

Her mother's experience had caused Lisa considerable anxiety whenever she had had a mammogram, a situation exacerbated when the staff would tell her to come back for a second look, which was not infrequent. Mammograms are a bit scattershot in reliability, but doctors will point out that in *most* breast cancer cases, it's the best tool we have right now.

Even so, Lisa's mother's experience was now playing another role—her mother had been stoic; she never had complained afterward; and she had survived. Lisa would be like her. She would fight.

In the operating room, Lisa arose from a stretcher and lay down on the operating table. She thought of the time when she and our son Danny, then about fourteen, were at Universal Studios Orlando, and she had felt weak and hollow, her hands shaking. Danny had rushed to get her a flavored ice drink then looked at her imploringly, hoping everything would be all right.

She started to cry. The anesthesiologist said, "Don't you worry! You're going to be fine. I'm going to take good care of you. Nothing bad is going to happen." Such kindness yet again. It was the last memory Lisa had before her disease-ridden body was subjected to the mother of all surgeries.

Three

Either the well was very deep, or she fell very slowly, for she had plenty of time as she went down to look about her and to wonder what was going to happen next –from Lewis Carroll's Alices's Adventures in Wonderland

Wednesday, the day after. In the intensive care unit, Lisa believed wrongly that she had awakened on the operating table. Although she heard activity and conversation, she could neither move nor speak and seemed to be looking out through a keyhole. *Oh, my God*, she thought. *Am I going to be one of those people who wakes up and can't tell them I'm awake, and they're going to start cutting into me, and it's going to be excruciating...?*

She drifted off again and later awoke in the middle of a conversation. The nurses were talking with her. Her whole body was bloated from the fluids that were necessary for the operation. One of her eyes was swollen shut, and the other was almost so. Her stomach was being drained through a tube in her nose. Multiple tubes ran from her abdomen, draining liquid into plastic bottles.

Her throat was parched. At some point her breathing tube was removed, and she asked for some ice. Though she was still heavily drugged, her recovery had begun.

If Lisa were told any details of her surgery, she wouldn't have remembered them. Harriet, the enterostomal therapy nurse, came to talk with her about her ostomy, but she had no memory of it.

Doctor Sardi had told Lisa that getting an ostomy was possible, even likely, in her case. Protruding from her abdomen was a swollen stoma, the consistency of which was similar to the inside cheeks of one's mouth. She later read somewhere that maintaining an ostomy was as routine as brushing one's teeth, and as time went on, she found that was true. At this time Harriet reassured her that various statesmen and celebrities had gotten along fine with ostomies.

She would be taken up to the fifteenth floor two days after surgery, but first her physical therapist made sure she walked the floor of the ICU on the very first day. This was standard practice for Doctor Sardi's patients and helped prevent an embolism, a potentially fatal blood clot.[1]

What is now Mercy Hospital began in 1870 as Baltimore City Hospital, a dispensary for the poor that was housed in an abandoned schoolhouse. Would-be doctors would undergo their training there. Shortly after the hospital opened, the Sisters of Mercy, then attending to sick and wounded Civil War veterans in Washington, DC, were asked to take over the facility. In 1909 Baltimore City Hospital became Mercy Hospital. Later it also served food to the poor during the Great Depression.

One urban legend regarding the hospital is that during the Great Baltimore Fire of 1904, while the Sisters of Mercy were attending to injured firemen in addition to their regular charges, the fire threatened to engulf the hospital, but concerted prayer caused the prevailing winds to change direction. Today's urban legend is yesterday's miracle.

The 1904 fire left an indelible stamp on the city. The city itself was rebuilt with $6 million in railroad profit. Most noticeably, stone or brick was mandated by law in subsequent buildings, resulting in the ubiquitous brick row homes or, as they are more likely to be called in today's gentrified neighborhoods, townhouses.

Today Baltimore Mercy Hospital is spread across four buildings, one of which is a parking garage. Once in any of the four buildings, one needn't take to the street, as the buildings are connected, two of them by second-story enclosed walkways. The walkway from the parking garage, which serves the Bunting Center, doubles as a sort of museum wing, with artifacts, short descriptions, and enlarged photographs on wall panels.

Facing the complex, the oldest building, in the center, is the McAuley Building; to the left, the Mary Catherine Bunting Center, opened in 2010; to the right, the Harry and Jeanette Weinberg Center, opened in 2003. In a city that was already a medical mecca of the New World, with the prestigious Johns Hopkins University Hospital, the University of Maryland Medical Center, and other renowned hospitals, Mercy, in spite of its humble origins, is now recognized as one of the best hospitals in the country.

Across from the Bunting Center and the McAuley Center is the narrow Preston Gardens Park, with fountains near each end.

There are staircases on each side of the fountains and a larger staircase in the center, all leading up to the northbound lane of Saint Paul Place. Adorning the park is a wide variety of flora and a dozen or so tables with chairs for dining, relaxing, or very occasional live music or poetry readings. Some tables sit in the shade; some have royal-blue umbrellas. At the left end of the park, again facing Saint Paul Place, is an unmarked black statue of Confederate general and railroad executive John Mifflin Hood, who was responsible for much of the money that rebuilt Baltimore after the 1904 fire. Surrounding the statue is a ring of evergreen shrubbery.

There is a story behind the names on each of the buildings.

The McAuley Center is named after the founder of the Sisters of Mercy, Catherine McAuley, an Irish woman who was inspired by the kind works of her father, who had died when she was five. She was taken in by another couple, and when she eventually came into an inheritance of what might now be considered about $2.7 million all told, she decided to commit her time and money to serving the poor.[2]

In the Catholic church, every day is a feast day, and in 1827, on the Feast of Our Lady of Mercy, September 24, the first residents, homeless and abused women, came to live in the House of Mercy on Baggot Street in Dublin. Two years later the chapel was dedicated.

The years in Ireland from about 1815 to 1850 were those of economic crisis, with causes ranging from waves of unemployed young men coming home from the Napoleonic Wars, to British import and export laws that made English goods valuable and Irish goods almost worthless. Poor sanitation in Dublin also contributed to the problem, leading to outbreaks of typhus, dysentery, and later cholera. The midcentury potato famine proved to be the straw that broke the camel's back. Though the potato rot existed throughout Europe, it hit Ireland the hardest, as many Irish lived on little else, with much of Ireland's other food products appropriated for needed income.

Catherine McAuley's work was intermittently controversial, even though she was more or less following in the footsteps of another Irish woman, Nano Nagle, who had founded the Presentation Sisters. In Nagle's time, a half century earlier, such work was outright illegal. Though the Sisters of Mercy are today better known worldwide, Nagle would still be the better known of the two in Ireland.

Part of the reason for the controversy was that McAuley opened the House of Mercy in one of Dublin's most affluent districts and continued to serve the poor during the time of cholera. When the Greek general and historian Thucydides (460 BC–395 BC), who first noticed that those who survive a plague are immune to it later, was himself stricken with plague, he was exiled. Readers of the New Testament are familiar with leper colonies. In medieval Europe, again, those stricken with plague were routinely exiled.

When McAuley died in 1841, there were 150 Sisters of Mercy; today there are thousands. Many of them are professional women; for example, a doctor at nearby Johns Hopkins, Dr. Karen Schneider, began as a Sister of Mercy and helped save a baby buried in the rubble after the 2010 Haitian earthquake.[3]

Before entering the McAuley Center, one passes a small garden with a winding flagstone path that leads to artist Marie Kullen's statue of McAuley, which was installed in 2000. Three flags—one for Baltimore, one for Maryland, and one for the United States, are hoisted above the revolving doors. Just beyond the revolving doors to the McAuley Center is the Catherine McAuley inscription:

In the care of the sick, great tenderness above all things...

At the age of sixteen, Mary Catherine Bunting, while a passenger in her boyfriend's car, was in a serious accident. The bones in her face were broken, and she spent ten days in the hospital with her mouth wired shut. Inspired by her nurses, she earned a nursing diploma from Mercy Hospital School of Nursing in 1958. She later earned a Bachelor of Arts degree from Mount Saint Agnes College, a Catholic college in the Mount Washington neighborhood of Baltimore that merged with Loyola College in 1972, and advanced degrees in nursing from the University of Maryland. She also received an honorary doctorate from Notre Dame of Maryland University in 2012.

Until 1996 she had a busy career, working as a nurse in labor and delivery, teaching, and becoming a nurse practitioner at Mercy Southern Health Center, which served the poor. She still remains reasonably busy as a volunteer.

In 1959 she joined the Sisters of Mercy, took the vows of poverty, and in so doing left a small fortune behind.

Mary Catherine Bunting's grandfather was George Avery Bunting, a former teacher and principal whose financial ambitions led him to leave education behind. He bought a drugstore in Baltimore in 1903. His earliest ambition, to market a liquid dental preparation, was abandoned with the introduction of toothpaste. His next experiment was with vanishing cream, what would now be called beauty cream. The first vanishing cream in the United States, introduced in 1892, was Hazeline Snow. Far more successful, however, was Pond's Vanishing Cream, introduced in 1904. Bunting took note.

His mother had used oil of cloves as a toothache remedy, so Bunting added this to his vanishing cream in 1914 to make Doctor Bunting's Sunburn Remedy. He later said, "...[I]f I could anesthetize the sunburned nerve endings long enough, nature would come along, and I would get the credit."

For years Bunting mixed small quantities of the stuff in a coffeepot in the back of his pharmacy, eventually pouring the remedy into small cobalt-blue glass jars. When a customer reported that the remedy had cured his eczema, had "knocked it right out," Noxzema was born.

As the country entered World War II, Noxzema was doing a little more than a million dollars in annual sales. The United States Army bought massive quantities of it for soldiers' tired feet, for insect bites, for jungle skin, for itching scalps, and even for shaving.[4] By the end of the war, annual sales had tripled.

That was the source of the small fortune Mary Catherine Bunting left behind.

The year after Mary Catherine took her vows of poverty, the Noxzema Company, now under the guidance of George Avery Bunting's son, George L. Bunting Sr., began to develop a modest collection of cosmetics called CoverGirl. In 1962 the company signed a sixteen-year-old model and sometime actress who already had been on the covers of *Vogue, Cosmopolitan,* and *Seventeen* to be their spokeswoman for the next thirty years. Her name was Jennifer O'Neill, and her signing, along with the signing of Cybill Shepherd in the late 1960s, Christie Brinkley in 1985, and numerous others, helped ensure that CoverGirl would become the top-selling makeup line in the United States.

In 1974 Mary Catherine Bunting no longer felt called by God to maintain her vows of poverty.[5] The fortune she had left behind was now much larger, and surely she realized that in addition to her nursing, her teaching, and her serving the poor, she could do a great deal of good as a philanthropist. Though the woman who was once a nun does not now live her life much differently than she ever did, she has supported a variety of projects generously and has given the largest donation in Mercy Hospital's history to the center that bears her name.

There are eight panels of translucent, colored stone pressed between sheets of sheer glass outside the Bunting Center. Here too is the start of a wall made of Jerusalem limestone, which extends to the entrance to the Chapel of Light, a place for prayer. Two stories of the brilliant panels make up the exterior wall of the chapel, while the limestone is also used in the spacious lobby.

A single candle in the chapel stands upon a pedestal of stunningly variegated green marble, and this same beautiful marble accents every floor in the building.

Two revolving doors mark the entrance of the Weinberg Center. At the far right end there is a panel of falling water that is straddled on either side by veined, translucent glass. On either side of the fountain are marble-floored staircases. The main floor is a myriad of marble patterns, with three oases of maroon and gray and cream carpeting with comfortable armchairs and sofas.

The lobby reaches the ceiling of the second floor. The same panels of veined glass that bookend the waterfall also form the buffer for the three sides of the balcony on the second floor. On the second floor is the entrance to the McGlannan Health Sciences Library, though most of the library is up a short flight of stairs within. On the same floor, to the left, is the Truman T. Semans Education and Conference Center, dedicated November 20, 2003.

The Harry and Jeanette Weinberg Foundation provided about one-fourth of the funding for the center that bears their name. In his lifetime Harry Weinberg could have inspired an Oliver Stone movie. He was born in 1908 in Galicia, then part of the Austro-Hungarian Empire, and at age four, he came to the United States. After spending nearly all of his school years in disciplinary classes, he dropped out in the sixth grade to work in his father's auto repair shop. During the Great Depression, he bought distressed Baltimore properties and later sold them at a profit. Prior to World War II, he bought massive amounts of automobile tires, also selling them at a profit. He was rich.

Weinberg retired at age forty in 1948 but became bored. Next came a string of successes in the transit business, beginning with a purchase of bonds in the Baltimore Transit Company. Later he controlled mass transit in Scranton, Pennsylvania; Dallas; Honolulu; and New York.

The New York acquisition, in 1962, just prior to the New York World's Fair, was the Fifth Avenue Coach Line, then the largest bus line in the world, though it was having financial difficulties. Weinberg attempted to double the ten-cent fare, but New York Mayor Robert Wagner scotched the plan. As a result, Weinberg began to lay off workers, causing a strike.[6] Wagner then went to the New York legislature for approval to buy out the bus line, eventually netting Weinberg thirty-two dollars per share for his twelve-dollar-per-share investment.[7]

Weinberg was hardly beloved in Baltimore. *Forbes* magazine consistently referred to him as "combative, aggressive, and litigious."[8] In the eighties, Baltimore mayor William Donald Schaefer, who later became governor of Maryland, asked Weinberg to fix some of the deteriorating sixty or so buildings that he owned in the downtown area. When Weinberg refused, Schaefer purportedly was livid. Some felt Weinberg preferred the $50 million tax write-off. Bernard Berkowitz, Baltimore's physical development coordinator at the time, said:

I enjoyed [talking with Weinberg], because I have a weakness for Damon Runyon characters. He'd talk in a kind of stream of consciousness, with sentences that didn't always have verbs...But this was a very difficult man to deal with, very fixed in his opinions and attitudes. He was very clear about what was the city's role and what was the private sector's role [in restoring the city].[9]

Weinberg's extreme thrift might also be partly explained by a comment made by a close friend of his, attorney Lawrence Weisman, who said that Weinberg always feared losing his fortune.[10]

In the fifties, with the advent of jet travel, Weinberg realized that Hawaii, a sleepy military outpost, would be accessible to the world. He bought huge, inexpensive tracts of land that later would be worth hundreds of millions. In 1959 he set up the Harry and Jeanette Weinberg Foundation. In 1968 he and his wife moved to Hawaii permanently. He had come to Baltimore as a street urchin who couldn't stay out of trouble. He could move to Hawaii as a demigod.

In 1984 Weinberg gave his critics a glimpse of things to come when he donated funds to air-condition all of Israel's nursing homes. Upon his death due to bone cancer in 1990, less than a year after the passing of his wife, he gave a substantial but undisclosed amount of money to his only son, $3 million to his grandchildren, and with the caveat that 25 percent of the rest be spent on Jewish charities, he gave almost $1 billion to the poor.

Lisa's days began at five thirty in the morning, sort of. She tried to sleep at night but sometimes lay awake for hours at a time. Conversely, during the day, whether she was propped up in her bed or propped up in the reclining armchair beside her bed, she would drift off any number of times. When it was light out, she could see downtown Baltimore through the large window in her room. When it was dark, she could see a sliver of light on the ceiling, as the door to her room was never completely shut. The days and nights blended together; five thirty was merely another visit to the room for the nursing assistant who was coming to take her vitals and to draw blood. Later there would be a faint glow from the window, a sign that dawn was breaking.

She had been fed intravenously for the first week or so. Her first attempt at eating had not gone well, so she needed to be fed intravenously again until her digestive system came back on line entirely. This was not an unusual complication for someone who had undergone a prolonged surgery and who had had the contents of her abdominal cavity rearranged.

All the pleasure of ingestion came from what she drank, which was water, apple juice, and cranberry juice. The fifteenth floor of the Bunting Center, where all of Doctor Sardi's patients recovered, was pretty well stocked with these items and other things, but Lisa had asked for extra to be brought in from a grocery store, just in case.

The assistant nurse was finished. Three or four elaborate bouquets, an orchid, and dozens of get-well cards were silhouetted on the shelf by the window. Lisa would drift back to sleep.

There was always some commotion around seven in the morning. The nurses worked twelve-hour shifts, so seven in the morning and seven in the evening were the changing of the guards. A nurse would come in, write his or her name on the board, and change the other information written on the board if necessary.

The physical therapist, whom Lisa referred to as "Miss Sonya," would wake her up. It was now completely light out, time for her to walk the perimeter of the fifteenth floor to build her strength and to prevent embolisms. Lisa dreaded this, but everyone told her it was necessary. It hardly mattered, as Miss Sonya would not take "no" from her, or any other patient, for that matter. At first, Lisa hated her and dreaded seeing her face in the doorway. She felt Miss Sonya was insensitive and oblivious to her pain and exhaustion. In Miss Sonya's eyes she was lazy and good for nothing. As the days went by and the effects of the drugs began to subside, Lisa became willing to concede that she was the tough-love type, ideal for the job.

The walks started out as a big production then got simpler as time went on. In the beginning Lisa had a half dozen catheters running from her body to small plastic bottles, collecting her fluids as they drained. They all would have to be pinned someplace or other. Her fluid pumps, clicking or beeping or both, were mounted on several levels of what looked like a hat rack on wheels and had to be unplugged, with all the cords wrapped up and out of the way. One person would help her with the hat rack, while another would push the reclining armchair, which, with a kick of a lever, glided right along behind her. Eventually she would ditch the catheters and the plastic bottles one by one and the chair as well.

This was the first of three, maybe four such daily excursions. During the course of the day, other patients moved slowly past Lisa's room, leaning on their hat racks, soldiering on. Even though her door was always open, she could pull what amounted to a shower curtain to one side so she could have some privacy, and all the people who passed would then become silhouettes.

When Lisa returned to her room, she would order breakfast. She had four or five categories and could pick one item from each. When she finally could tolerate solids, she ate only a small fraction of her food, though her appetite would later increase. Lunch and dinner also had menu choices.

Lisa's job was to recover; it would consume all her energy and resources. Around her were accoutrements and toys that would help her through the process. One of the first things she had been told to do was to put her feet on the floor and move them back and forth. She looked down at her yellow socks that had a multitude of small white pieces of latex or something, modeled after paramecium maybe, and designed to prevent slippage. This exercise helped prevent deep venous thrombosis, embolisms. She had something to squeeze over and over, first with one hand then with the other. She also had an incentive spirometer; she could blow into it and get the little blue ball to rise to the top, something to help prevent pneumonia. She also had equipment she never used, such as a device to help put on socks and another that vaguely resembled a caulking gun, designed for grabbing things several feet away.

During the time she had been fed intravenously, she didn't have to think much about her ostomy. Now that Lisa had begun to eat solids, Harriet, the ostomy nurse, would work with her on the maintenance. Every room on the fifteenth floor was a private room with a private bath, which made things easier.

I had taken an extended leave from teaching, without pay, and would show up between ten and ten thirty in the morning. I spent the first two or three hours of my day doing light remodeling at our home—painting the rooms, refinishing the floors, outfitting the bathroom for safety, running cable up to the second floor, and so on. I read Lisa any new cards or mail and offered to read her e-mail. I would usually leave about six thirty, sometimes after Marcy visited, sometimes before.

Whenever Lisa left the fifteenth floor, she would wait for someone from the transport department to get her into a wheelchair and push her to the main nurses' station. There she would pick up a binder that documented all her whereabouts and all her procedures. It eventually would be as thick as a major metropolitan telephone directory. Sometimes I would carry it along; sometimes Lisa held it in her lap. Wherever she stopped, transport would leave and would have to be called back when she was ready for the next stop. Sometimes transport came quickly; sometimes they took a long time. Months after Lisa was released, someone in the hospital put up a big board in the middle of the McAuley Center with the names of all the transport employees on it, ranking them in terms of their average time per mission completed. After that first month, the rankings were taped on the door of the nurses' office between the McAuley Center and the Bunting Center. After that the rankings disappeared.

Sometimes Lisa's transport person would cheer her up. When she bemoaned her seemingly endless hospital stay, one young woman said in a voice deliberately made to sound conspiratorial, "I can get you to the front door. After that you're on your own."

The fifteenth floor was laid out like a digital number eight, with the nurses' station in the middle. There also were two sets of elevators, one for medical personnel and visitors, one for medical personnel and patients. The hospital was labyrinthine in nature, at least partly as a matter of security. Transport in the early days was to specialists' offices. In a few days, Lisa also would be starting occupational therapy downstairs.

Only a few days earlier, there had been a sign on her door that had read, NEUTROPENIA. Her white blood cell count was so low that the room had been quarantined; everyone who came in and out had to wear a mask. It was not an unusual complication for patients who had been subjected to HIPEC, but now the sign was down, and the door was wide open again.

In addition to the nurse's assistants, who took her vitals every four hours, Lisa would see the nurse who was scheduled to supervise her room that day; she had two favorite nurse, both named Leah, one of whom was studying for her master's degree at Johns Hopkins. On any given day, other visitors included Doctor Sardi's physician assistants, Nick Athas and Stephanie Lackey; his administrative assistant, Jennifer Francis; Sardi himself; and occasionally his colleague, Doctor Vadim Gushchin.

Jennifer Francis had started in Doctor Sardi's office compiling data on his patients. Prior to her arrival, the data had been collected retrospectively, depending on the purpose of the research paper at hand. She had built a database that would keep track of all factors and would follow the patients year after year. When the position of HIPEC coordinator opened up, she did both jobs for a while. For many patients she was their primary connection; if someone were overwhelmed or were having money worries, he or she might feel more comfortable talking to her than to a clinician. Helping people whenever she could was her favorite part of the job.

Late in the afternoon, Doctor Sardi came to visit Lisa. During the brief chat, he said, in a magnanimous voice that contrasted sharply with the seriousness of the subject matter, "You need to start walking, my friend! Or you will die!"

This rattled Lisa. She thought she had been doing her walking. But she often had skipped that fourth walk, stretching three of them out until Miss Sonya, Marcy, and I had gone home. Doctor Sardi again emphasized that Lisa needed to avoid an embolism, and that fourth walk was an important part of the process.

Shortly after I left, Marcy came. She had come every day so far and would continue to come every day, except for the week when she went to a conference. Sometimes her duties as a doctor caused her to come rather late, leaving Lisa to wonder whether she were ever coming at all. Good day or bad day, Lisa was always glad to see her.

Marcy grew up in Edgerton, Wisconsin, a town of four thousand that had one traffic light. In her childhood Edgerton celebrated Tobacco Days; now they celebrate Heritage Days. Marcy went off to college as a prospective first-grade teacher, which she saw as a little better fit for her than the two other occupations expected of Edgerton girls—secretary or nurse. College proved liberating; for the first time, she could admit she liked science and math, and she began to prepare to be a medical technician. Even so, it wasn't until her junior year when she learned in a casual conversation that another girl was a premed major. When Marcy realized her own grades were better than the premed major's, she decided to find out what it would take to get into medical school. Nothing ventured, nothing gained. She was one of eleven women among 121 students in her graduating class at the Medical College of Wisconsin in Milwaukee.

She later would accompany a mentor, Doctor George Weilis, to Africa under the auspices of the group Médecins Sans Frontières, better known in the United States as Doctors Without Borders. Later she also would accompany Doctor Armando Sardi on a mission to Cali, Colombia.

With Médecins Sans Frontières, Doctor Marcella Roenneberg, a nationally recognized expert in urinary incontinence and pelvic reconstructive surgery, traveled to Niger, Sierra Leone, and Bangladesh, treating women who had vesicovaginal fistulas, holes between the bladder and vagina, which led to uncontrolled urination. In the United States, surgeons could repair these tears when they occurred during the natural course of childbirth. In Africa these women were the untouchables, often abandoned by their husbands and ostracized by their communities. Marcy has healed scores of such women over the years.

Stephanie Lackey, one of Doctor Sardi's three physician assistants who also had attended to her surgery, was assigned to Lisa's care. Stephanie is a quiet and compassionate woman who works with lithe, catlike precision. Lisa looked forward to her many visits, and the patient-caregiver bond that had been developing between the two was especially strengthened on the day Stephanie first removed Lisa's nasogastric tube. In spite of the medical protocol that Lisa's digestive system *should* have been ready at this point, it was not, and Stephanie had to thread the tube back down the esophagus at a time when Lisa's every instinct was to gag. A near panic quickly became a shared relief.

Massive surgeries such as the one Lisa underwent almost always result in minor complications, though not always the same minor complications. In general the white blood cell count decreases until day twelve. In general the digestive system comes back on line between days four and six. In general diarrhea can be expected until day twelve. In general the nasogastric tube, which runs from the nose to the stomach, comes out around day six. In Lisa's case she was also treated for a fever and a urinary tract infection, neither of which was unusual. There were times when she suggested to the medical staff that she was somehow making a nuisance of herself, but Stephanie and others were always quick to reassure her that this simply was not true.

It was mid-September, now getting dark around seven, and the descending darkness was the hardest time for Lisa. She would read a little, rest a little, watch a little TV. Mostly because of the drugs, she had difficulty following or staying awake for a whole TV show, but Mercy Hospital had a channel which showed only landscapes set to soothing music. The landscapes were in a loop, and Lisa waited for the tropical beach. She imagined that it was in Thailand and all the people there lived carefree lives. She promised herself that if she pulled through she would go there someday.

Her cell phone had disappeared, so she was resigned to taking calls on the phone in her room, assuming her would-be callers knew she was in this particular hospital. The loss of her cell phone was only a small financial burden, as it was an older model, but she deeply regretted not having downloaded years of photos to some other source. They would be lost forever.

She had, understandably, been dwelling on the subject of death lately. Her old life was slipping away. The idea of getting out of bed, showering, getting dressed and going to work as a strategic planner seemed a bit more surreal with each passing day. She missed Danny. She missed our pets. She missed her old life.

It was hard on her now, but it probably had been even a little harder that first week. The nurses always asked her, "On a scale of one to ten, how would you describe your pain?" Her answer was almost always "One" or "Two." She had been on powerful, psychotropic drugs. Medication was pumped continually to her incision. She had a little hand pump that all patients in a similar situation get, designed so that overdosing is not possible; she could push the button with her thumb if anything started to hurt, so pain wasn't much of an issue for her.

Anxiety was the main issue. She would need her pillow propped up a bit because her neck was getting a bit sore, but she could not yet do it herself. She would ring for the nurse, hoping someone, anyone, would come. Her mouth was parched, and she needed a cup of ice. The questions that arose were troubling. What would her life be like now? Would the cancer come back? What if she were to die? What if she were to die in this very room?

Lisa drifted off to sleep.

In the morning her gaze wandered over to the portable table by her bed. There was the latest copy of *Entertainment Weekly*, a small green box of facial tissue, her incentive spirometer, and a cup partially filled with melted ice. There was also something new; in a slender vase was a single red rose, compliments of Doctor Armando Sardi.

Early in his life, it would not have been unfair to character-ize Armando Sardi as a hopelessly romantic man, even if such an image conjured up nothing more than Don Quixote tilting at windmills. Today it would be fairer to characterize him as an incurably passionate man. He tells his two daughters, "If you're going to dance, it has to be like the last time you're going to do it! If you're going to kiss someone, kiss them like it's the last time you will ever kiss them!"

The city in which he grew up, Santiago de Cali, Colombia, is located in one of the richest valleys in the world. Cali also sits on the Pacific Ring of Fire; the city is surrounded not only by mountains, but also volcanoes. The area has a tropical climate; throughout the year the fluctuations in the weather are very mi-nor. If one goes into the mountains only twenty minutes away, the weather becomes colder rather abruptly, and snow can be seen on the mountaintops year round. It is around the rim of the valley and in the mountains that the poorest people live, the very people for whom Doctor Sardi became instrumental in improving health services.

Armando Sardi was one of seven children. In grade school he was fond of mathematics, calculus, and physics. Until about two months before he graduated, he assumed he would become an engineer.

In those days a college degree was offered in only four areas: law, architecture, engineering, and medicine. If you wanted to be a psychologist or philosopher, for example, you could put up your shingle and do so, but you wouldn't make a living at it. Today a wider choice of options is available.

Abruptly switching career tracks and passing the test to get into medical school, Armando found himself with a gestation period before he could attend Universidad del Valle, due to student unrest and violence that was occurring at the time. It was suggested that he go to the United States for a while to learn English. A Catholic family in the small town of Mosinee, Wisconsin, adopted him and treated him like a son. Some people in Mosinee knew nothing of Colombia, so he was fond of perpetuating their illusions, talking of sleeping in the trees and trying to get used to wearing clothing.

During his time in Mosinee, Armando would talk to his American mother about accomplishing many things in life then getting married at the age of thirty-five. She apparently knew him better than that, betting him twenty-five dollars that he would be married within five years. When he did marry a few years later, his American parents came to his wedding in Cali. Armando's Colombian father reciprocated the gesture by adopting the American daughter for the summer so the Sardi family could show her all of Colombia.

Over the past thirty years, the Sardi family has experienced more than its share of kidnappings. In one instance Armando's mother and brother were kidnapped; in another, a different brother. In his extended family, an uncle and a cousin have been kidnapped. The Sardis count themselves fortunate, as the immediate family members were rescued in both cases before being ransomed or killed, and although members of the extended family had to be ransomed, they arrived home safely. In Colombia kidnappings are much more common than they are in the United States. *Anyone* can get kidnapped if they wander from the beaten path, though the country is safer today than it was a generation ago, when the drug cartels were more powerful. Some kidnappings are political, but most are purely for profit.

When Armando was ready for college, Colombia did not have separate graduate and postgraduate degrees but instead offered a European-style program. For Armando this meant seven years of medical school, including a rotating internship. Although the Colombian tuition system was based on family need, he was able to improve on that by getting a full scholarship for two of those years, once for finishing first in his class and once for finishing second. The extra money proved useful, as at this point, he may have been the only one in medical school who was married and had a child.

In Colombia the last year in medical school is spent doing rural duty. Doctor Sardi has fond memories of his time on San Andrés Island, a Colombian island off the coast of Nicaragua, though there was sadness too. One night when he was on call, his wife came to him distraught, barefoot, and soaking wet from having jumped into a pool. His first thought was that someone had died, but he did not know yet that it was his own son,

Mauricio, who had drowned in a pool among ten people or so, none of whom initially noticed he was missing. Armando and his wife went to where the body lay, in an incubator that had been used as a last attempt at resuscitation. There was nothing for Armando to do now but wrap up the slender remains in a blanket and carry them home. He took two days off from work then declared to his wife that since another baby was on the way, the child needed to be brought into a happy home.

In recalling the event, Doctor Sardi does not speak of it so much in terms of how the boy's life was taken away but how lucky he was to have had those precious few years with him, an outlook not uncommon among people of faith. Even so, he says he misses Mauricio more now than when he first lost him, when every door in the world was potentially wide open to him and he was still only twenty-five.

Lisa's therapy now included an hour or more in the occupational therapy room downstairs. Transport would wheel her down to the reception area, where the thick book that documented her entire stay was handed off to the nurse at the reception desk. There was usually a short wait until the next therapist was available, and generally four or five therapists were working with individual patients. The therapists introduced themselves and chatted with the patients to find out how they were doing before any activity was undertaken.

It was a large, cheerful room, functional in nature. There was a bed to practice getting in and out of and a shower stall for the same purpose. Many patients simply walked.

There also was a partial staircase, which was usually occupied. In Lisa's case and probably in many cases, mastering the stairs was necessary before a patient was released from the hospital. Because patients were often still on pain medication, the activity could be dangerous.

Often the activities practiced here were rudimentary, such as working with buttoned clothing. Lisa had to renegotiate such basics because of her partial neuropathy. Of course, for patients who had lost limbs, what was basic was by no means easy, especially at first. Though this was not true for Lisa, patients who are debilitated often need to consider another line of work entirely, and some will not be able to work at all.

Among the therapies specific to Lisa's situation were gliding exercises. The long operation had left her with partial neuropathy, or loss of sensation, in her hands and fingers. The purpose of the gliding exercises—the twisting of the wrists and stretching of the fingers that were reminiscent of yoga—was to regain sensation. She later would continue these exercises at home, recovering complete sensation after about four and a half months.

After sixteen days Lisa was discharged. The topmost leaves on the trees in front of our house were just now turning yellow.

Her blood pressure and cholesterol levels were normal, and she no longer had elevated blood-sugar counts. She was taken off Crestor, metformin and Lisinopril, drugs she had taken for years that she probably would not need again.[11] She was, however, still being treated for a bladder infection, not an unusual complication for someone who had had to use a urinary catheter temporarily. She also was prescribed medicine for her pain and her anxiety, which she used sparingly, as well as a blood thinner. The blood thinner caused uncontrollable nose bleeding after about six days, necessitating an overnight trip to the emergency room.

Lisa's main job, so to speak, would continue to be what it had been—to recuperate. She kept up her walking schedule but mostly rested or watched TV. She always had been an avid reader of books, and she eventually resumed that habit as well.

Her diet included oatmeal, Cream of Rice, macaroni and cheese, and prepared peaches and pears. For about a month she couldn't swallow or was afraid to swallow. She eventually moved on to such things as turkey sandwiches.

I became a full-time caregiver, on duty at all times. Around the fourth or fifth day, I had taken our dog on a walk, and Lisa had expected me back in ten or fifteen minutes. When I wasn't back, she called me on my cell phone.

I sounded angry. I said that if she were to call me again when I was walking our pet, and it wasn't an emergency, I would hang up on her. Lisa felt bad. She didn't like being helpless. She didn't like having to depend on others. It wasn't her fault that she couldn't do everything for herself.

By the time I returned, I had realized I had been nothing but a bully. I apologized profusely, remarking that although she had been the one who had been prescribed anxiety medicine, maybe I was the one who should have been taking it. There's a cautionary tale in here somewhere about trying to become a round-the-clock, seven-days-a-week caregiver overnight, with little or no relief from friends and family.

In 1987 Doctor Sardi, who was on a fellowship at Ohio State University, was awarded an American Cancer Society Fellowship Grant to do research. His interest at the time was in using a handheld gamma detector in the diagnosis of colon cancer. As the gold standard for any diagnostic technique is that all patients who test positive have the condition, while all patients who test negative do not have the condition, Sardi's procedure ultimately generated too many false positives to be useful in that application. Later, however, the concept was applied with greater success to cases of melanoma and breast cancer, and today the use of the handheld gamma detector is a standard option in hospitals.

During that year Doctor Sardi had the chance to work with Doctor John Peter Minton, a man who, like Sardi, had a passion for everything in which he became involved. He was a surgeon who used aggressive surgery to treat cases of colorectal cancer that other surgeons wouldn't touch. He was sometimes in surgery for extended periods.

Prior to his year at Ohio State with Doctor Minton, Doctor Sardi hardly would have believed these protracted surgeries were possible. Although Sardi considered the surgical technique he had learned in Colombia and at Saint Agnes quite good, he was able to enhance it further under Minton, who had developed the technique for removing tumors that had spread from the colon to the liver and that previously had been considered inoperable. Today this technique sometimes is called the Swiss cheese operation. Minton began in 1977 by removing a few lesions then progressively became more aggressive in subsequent surgeries.[12]

Doctor Minton passed away following a car accident he had on his way to work in 1990. He was only fifty-six. Befitting his status as a champion rosarian, his widow, Janice, donated a rose garden with thirty varieties of roses set like jewels among other woody and herbaceous plants, to Ohio State University, and the garden is still maintained today. In 2002 the city of Upper Arlington, Ohio, recognized him with a bronze plaque on its Wall of Honor.

Four

With purity and with holiness I will pass my life and practice my Art. --from the Hippocratic Oath

Doctor Armando Sardi's search for a position in the United States is a study in persistence. After his stay in Mosinee, Wisconsin, he decided he would return to the States after finishing medical school in Colombia, and his wife, who was willing to stay behind with their daughters for two weeks, encouraged him to fulfill his ambition. In order to return, he took and passed a medical exam and the Visa Qualifying Exam (VQE). With two pieces of luggage, two letters of introduction, and some seed money, he took a flight to Miami and began his search for a program where he could be a surgical resident, a keenly competitive position.

An anesthesiologist in Miami told him there was no way that in early June he would get into a surgical residency program that would start July 1, especially with a mere letter, and he invited Doctor Sardi to work with him for a year as a house officer in a hospital. This would place him in a position to later get training in a specialty, Sardi's real ambition.

Some people would be satisfied with such an offer, but the young Sardi deferred an acceptance, sat alone on a Miami boulevard, dejected, and thought through his options. Though there is no such thing as a year that is truly lost, from his point of view, life was too precious for him to be set back an entire year this way. He later called a Doctor Raskin from Baltimore, whom he had met while Raskin was visiting Colombia. Raskin told him he would call two local hospitals on his behalf. Sardi was aware that people had difficulty understanding him, especially on the phone, and, combining that awareness and his mother's adage, *the face of a saint makes the miracle*, he informed Raskin that he would not *call* the hospitals, but would instead fly to Baltimore.

He visited the Miami anesthesiologist, turned down the job, and flew to Baltimore, arriving on a rainy Friday night. The driver of the airport shuttle stopped several blocks before Sardi's destination, the Howard Street Hotel. It was the company's policy not to go farther than that, but Sardi, emphasizing the pouring rain, managed to talk him into it. The receptionist at the hotel was behind a sheet of bulletproof glass, and the door to his room had more locks on it than he had ever seen. When he tried to deposit money in a bank the next day, after having mentioned he was staying at the Howard Hotel, they refused to accept it.

On Monday he called Saint Agnes and South Baltimore, known as Harbor Hospital today. Saint Agnes had no openings, and South Baltimore told him that his certificates were not signed and that it could take up to a year for the Colombia Ministry of Health to sign them.

He returned to South Baltimore the next day, Tuesday, which puzzled the program director considerably. Sardi had rented a car, had driven to the Educational Commission for Foreign Medical Graduates in Philadelphia, and had convinced a senior administrator to sign a six-month temporary certificate. When the program director at South Baltimore saw the certificate, he was impressed enough with Sardi's pluck to say, "We had *better* hire you." He offered Sardi an observership position, but Sardi explained that he had a wife and two daughters and would need a paid position. He was then hired as a surgical resident and entered the five-year program.

In those days there may have been up to twenty candidates in the program, but only two of the incoming interns would be promoted to the second year. Many of those incoming freshman only needed one year of general surgery before moving on to their subspecialty anyway, but others would be disappointed at being cut from the program. Nowadays the students most likely to move up are designated from the very beginning, and the other interns know in advance that they'll have to move on unless something happens to open up.

The surgical residency program at South Baltimore was canceled in the middle of Doctor Sardi's second year and would become effective at the end of his fourth year. The idea behind the cuts was to downsize the surgical-residency programs in the United States from 450 to 250 centers.

This left Doctor Sardi, and for that matter, all students in their second year of residency at the centers being downsized, in an awkward position. It would be almost impossible to get into another program at the end of his fourth year, still needing one more year. He felt he needed to act before the second year was up.

While still at South Baltimore during that second year, the young Sardi applied to some of the most prestigious hospitals in the country. At one the interviewer, a gastrointestinal surgeon, turned his back on him. After some idle chatter, Sardi was told bluntly that the hospital didn't take foreigners. Sardi challenged him—what if he had flown all the way from South America just to hear that? The interviewer said simply that it was politics, so Sardi left.

Eventually the staff at South Baltimore implored Doctor John Singer of Saint Agnes Hospital in Baltimore to talk to Sardi, which led to his spending his last three years of residency there. Though Sardi started at Saint Agnes as an unknown, he would leave two decades later as an internationally renowned surgeon.

Doctor Singer belonged to a cadre of general surgeons who were diversified. He graduated from the SUNY medical school in Brooklyn, then served a two-year residency at the Tufts-New England Medical Center before moving on to the University of Maryland Hospital and later Saint Agnes. He performed a variety of operations, including gallbladder surgery; appendix, thyroid, parathyroid, and breast surgery; hemorrhoid surgery; and so on. As an intern he worked 110 to 120 hours per week, far more than the number allowed by law today. He recalled an old saying, an admonishment, really—"If you are only on call every other night, you're missing half the cases."

One of the highlights of his career was making a film for Saint Agnes that helped teach incoming medical professionals how to handle difficult situations. For example, in the film a black doctor is introduced to an elderly white woman, who insists someone else examine her. Doctor Singer mostly used volunteer interns and nurses while making the film but hired a few actors as well.

Doctor Singer recalls that the young Sardi graduated from the Saint Agnes program as one of its stars; he was very hard-working, intelligent, and personable. In addition to the training Doctor Sardi received under his tutelage, Singer feels Sardi's experience in Ohio and in New Orleans, as well as a year he spent setting up an oncology unit in Scotland, were all valuable. Had he stuck to gallbladder or breast surgery, Sardi might only be known as an excellent surgeon. But Sardi's adopting HIPEC when the procedure was still in its infancy, or perhaps toddler-hood, helped ensure an international reputation.

For all intents and purposes, there is no real controversy in treating PMP, appendiceal cancer, or epithelial mesothelioma, a rare cancer of the peritoneum, with HIPEC. Many, perhaps most, centers that don't do HIPEC refer their patients in these cases to an institution that does do HIPEC. The controversy arises from all the *other* cancers that are treated by HIPEC. For every case of PMP, there are ten cases of ovarian cancer and one hundred cases of colon cancer. If HIPEC were to become a widespread viable option for good candidates with those cancers, the number of HIPEC procedures in the United States could increase more than six times, from 1,500 per year to 10,000 per year.[1]

In 2011 Doctor Paul Sugarbaker was asked to debate at the American Society of Clinical Oncologists (ASCO) 2011 annual meeting, cited by *Good Morning America* as the Super Bowl of cancer professionals, and held each year in early June at McCormick Place on Lake Michigan, just south of Soldier Field in Chicago. At the time, of the four major cancer centers in the country, only one did HIPEC. Memorial Sloan-Kettering in New York, Johns Hopkins in Baltimore, and the Mayo Clinic in Rochester, Minnesota did *not* do HIPEC. MD-Andersen in Houston, Texas, *did* do HIPEC, but only for patients with appendiceal cancer. Even with the caveat that MD-Andersen treated appendiceal cancer with HIPEC, there was, at that time, no treatment for appendiceal cancer listed whatsoever with either the American Cancer Society or the National Comprehensive Cancer Network.

Doctor Sugarbaker debated Doctor David P. Ryan of the Harvard Medical School and Massachusetts General Hospital Cancer Center in Boston, though the debate was confined to metastatic colorectal cancer. Because the number of HIPEC procedures could increase dramatically if the use of HIPEC were widely accepted, there was obviously far more at stake than the credibility or the persuasiveness of Sugarbaker and Ryan. The debate wasn't really to be won or lost on the floors of the ASCO conference, but, at least partly, in the individual offices of insurance companies around the country, where decisions regarding which procedures will be covered are often made.[2]

In his brief overview, Doctor Ryan pointed out that proponents and detractors of HIPEC likened the current environment to different historical references in cancer treatment. Those who supported HIPEC could point to the work of Doctor Sugarbaker, Doctor John Peter Minton, and other pioneers who proved that colon cancer that had metastasized to the liver still could be treated surgically, in spite of widespread skepticism at the time. Detractors of HIPEC likened it to "the use of high-dose chemotherapy with autologous stem cell support in patients with breast cancer,"[3] more commonly known as "bone-marrow transplants," a promising treatment that, after fifteen randomized, controlled trials, showed no significant overall survival benefit.[4]

In expressing such caution, one important caveat should be kept in mind—most, if not all, of the high hopes surrounding this bone-marrow transplant procedure were based on the astounding published results of a South African doctor named Werner Bezwoda, whose work could not be duplicated elsewhere and that later proved fraudulent.[5] HIPEC, on the other hand, was practiced at the time in about two hundred centers worldwide, with a plethora of reports of success from dozens of centers, so the analogy barely fits, if it fits at all.

In fairness to Dr. Ryan, several of his concerns were legitimate, but some of those legitimate concerns could address the skill of the surgeon or protocols used in the past, rather than current protocols or the legitimacy of the procedure itself.

Doctor Ryan concluded his presentation with both a harsh assessment of the evidence to date and an announcement that a Phase III randomized trial might settle the matter.

Many patients are already enduring this costly, potentially harmful, therapy with no understanding of whether it truly is helping them live longer or feel better. Thankfully, a randomized study by the Walter Reed Army Medical Center and the American College of Surgeons evaluating cytoreductive surgery and HIPEC compared with standard chemotherapy is currently underway. A prospective, randomized clinical trial is the only way to answer the question.[6]

This was the trial we were introduced to in chapter one. Though the trial was designed for 328 patients, only one signed up. After eighteen months, the plug was pulled on the entire project on January 17, 2012. It doesn't appear that Doctor Ryan ever will get the randomized study he once insisted upon.

Does it matter? Or rather *should* it matter?

It is something of an oddity that the same man, Bradford Hill, who once saved science from one theoretical straitjacket has, probably without ever intending to, put science in another one. In 1884 the famed microbiologist Robert Koch established three rules for determining cause: the catalyst had to be present in a diseased being; it had to be isolated; and then it had to be present again when introduced to a secondary host. These rules worked well for infectious diseases—a tsetse fly bite could cause sleeping sickness; a mosquito bite could cause malaria; and so on.

By the mid twentieth century, it was abundantly clear to many that the then fifteen-fold increase in lung cancer could be attributed to smoking tobacco, but the notion of "cause" proved elusive. Mice could have their backs painted with tobacco tar daily and develop cancer, but the tobacco industry could counter that most people do not paint their backs with thick layers of tobacco tar each and every day. Of the many individuals who were interested in breaking out of Koch's straitjacket, Bradford Hill—the same Bradford Hill who decided doctors could not be trusted and developed the first randomized, controlled trial to establish a cure for TB—came up with a more expansive definition of cause that could be applied to maladies that were not infectious. He developed a list of correlations, no one of which was crucial to establishing cause but taken together would do so. Once Hill's criteria became established, doctors could bluntly tell their patients that smoking causes cancer, with no fear of reprisal from the tobacco companies.

Doctor Sugarbaker already had established cytoreductive surgery and HIPEC for appendiceal cancer and peritoneal mesothelioma without a clinical trial. The type of liver resections Doctor John Peter Minton and Sugarbaker had been doing since the 1970s also had been established without a clinical trial. There were plenty of other examples.

Because the thyroid gland absorbs nearly all the iodine in the bloodstream, two types of thyroid cancer, papillary thyroid cancer and follicular thyroid cancer, are treated with radioactive iodine after the thyroid is removed. The long-term prognosis for both is excellent when diagnosed in the early stages, with a five-year survival rate of almost 100 percent.[7] No clinical trial.

In 1970 only 10 percent of testicular cancer patients survived. In 1980 that figure had risen to an 80-percent survival rate; by 1990, 85 percent; and today, 95 percent. It is the highest cure rate ever for an adult malignancy, mainly because of a single chemotheraupetic drug, cisplatin, that was first synthesized in 1844. After cisplatin proved effective on rat sarcomas in 1969, Doctor Lawrence Einhorn of the Indiana University School of Medicine, in 1973, mixed the drug with two other agents to produce remarkable results, and subsequent trials merely fine-tuned the combinations.[8] No clinical trial.

In 2003 the R. Adams Shock Trauma Center in Baltimore teased out one factor retrospectively in the treatment of shock for 15,534 patients, finding that those who had received blood transfusions were almost three times more likely to die, and more than three times more likely to be admitted to the intensive care unit, than those who did not. The practice of routinely transfusing blood, except in instances in which extreme blood loss necessitated the practice, abruptly ended.[9] No clinical trial.

In 2003, also, a panel of experts representing eleven international organizations collaborated to develop a protocol for treating sepsis, more commonly called blood poisoning, with the use of antibodies being central to the protocol. Instead of a trial, they began with a modified Delphi method, in which a wide range of treatments is solicited from the group then culled by means of consensus.[10] Again no clinical trial.

In addition to the possibility of solving a medical problem through something akin to a modified Delphi method, a 2007 British article suggested a methodology to determine when a randomized trial might be considered unnecessary in the future. This methodology consisted of a wide signal-to-noise ratio, in which the signal is the treatment effect and the noise is the natural course of the condition.[11]

In the future there surely will be other instances when a randomized, controlled study will not be possible. Because the establishment of these protocols is so important for insurance purposes, the modified Delphi system, the signal-to-noise ratio, or something else entirely could pave the way for more patients to opt for HIPEC, or for that matter, any promising therapy.

A lot has happened in the two years since the Sugarbaker-Ryan debate. Memorial Sloan-Kettering now has a HIPEC program. So does Doctor David Ryan's own stomping grounds, Massachusetts General Hospital Cancer Center. In 2013 Doctor Sugarbaker remarked that worldwide acceptance of cytoreduction and HIPEC was happening much more quickly than he had expected.[12]

Nine days after the debate, Doctor Sugarbaker gave a presentation at a symposium in Washington, D.C. Doctor Sardi also gave a presentation, during which he discussed the complicated case of a patient of his who had undergone three HIPEC surgeries. No consensus was reached among the oncologists on hand regarding how the treatment should have gone, and Sardi presented the updated version of the case again in Berlin, Germany in late 2012. In 2007 the patient had been diagnosed with appendiceal cancer at age thirty-three. One of the chemotherapeutic agents used in the HIPEC, mytomycin C, had failed completely, so in a subsequent operation Sardi turned to melphalan, which worked very well. Sardi described it as being especially good for high-resistant tumors, while Sugarbaker called it a very powerful drug. Apparently they were the only two oncologists at that symposium who used melphalan for HIPEC, and Sugarbaker suggested they publish their findings. It was an incidental exchange, all things considered.

Less than three months later, melphalan was the only agent used for Lisa's HIPEC.

Cisplatin. Mytomycin C. Melphalan. Where do they get this stuff?

About half an hour before midnight on Dec 2, 1943, 105 German bombers, having achieved complete surprise, descended upon the port city of Bari, located on Italy's east coast. In less than an hour, twenty-eight vessels were sunk, and twelve others were damaged. Among them was the American ship SS *John Harvey,* which, apparently unbeknownst to its own crew, contained seventy tons of mustard gas, an insidious poison. It was said that windows shattered up to seven miles away when the ship exploded. At the time one thousand casualties were reported, with an unknown number of additional casualties in the following months due to exposure to the gas.

The United States War Department issued no statement for two weeks; there was no mention of the mustard gas in *The New York Times* or the *Washington Post* that year, or for any number of years afterward; and a top-secret project was accelerated to investigate the effects of poisonous wartime gases on humans.[13] The contract for studying mustard gas in particular had been given to scientists Louis Goodman and Alfred Gilman of Yale University. A good place for them to have started would have been the writings of Edward Bell Krumbhaar, an American army captain who had treated soldiers exposed to mustard gas during World War I.

The first gas used in warfare had been chlorine, but because of its yellowish-green appearance, soldiers learned to avoid it. Then mustard gas was used, which was difficult to detect until one was immersed in it and confronted by its powerful odor. Captain Krumbharr had had a chance to examine thirty-four survivors of a mustard-gas attack, which he referred to at the time as "Yello[w] Cross Gas," as the shells that delivered the gas were each marked with a yellow cross. He derived a white blood cell count by looking at blood samples in a ten-by-ten-micron grid under a microscope, then extrapolated that to the standard measure, cells per cubic milliliter. Whereas a healthy white blood cell count would be in the range of four thousand to eleven thousand, these soldiers had counts well below one thousand, with some counts close to zero, a condition known as leucopenia. Captain Krumbharr suggested, "If anything would ever help these men, it would be some treatment to replenish their white [blood] cells." A researcher subsequently performed a comprehensive study of the effects of mustard gas on twenty-seven rabbits, confirming Krumbharr's observation.[14]

Goodman and Gilman began to think about the problem backward. If mustard gas were so effective at *killing* white bloods cells, could this poison instead be used to treat leukemia, a cancer of *runaway* white blood cell counts? This would not be the first attempt to find a cure for cancer, but it did represent a paradigm shift.

In fact the term *chemotherapy* was coined by German chemist and 1908 Nobel Prize winner Paul Ehrlich in the early 1900s, and it initially applied mostly to drugs used to fight infectious diseases. Ehrlich was a friend of Robert Koch, the man who defined "cause" for infectious diseases. Ehrlich, along with his colleagues, had had notable success in the treatment of syphilis and diphtheria, the latter treatment inspiring 1925's *Great Race of Mercy*. Ehrlich also was interested in testing drugs to fight cancer but was not optimistic about the prospects. Over the door to the cancer lab was a sign: GIVE UP ALL HOPE OH YE WHO ENTER.[15]

A few years after Ehrlich won his Nobel Prize, George Clowes of Roswell Park Memorial Institute in Buffalo, New York, where Mercy's Doctor Vadim Gushchin would apprentice nearly a century later, developed the first transplantable tumor system in rodents. Now an almost infinite array of substances could be tested for the treatment of cancer. Initial progress, however, was excruciatingly slow. Biochemist Murray Shear led testing at what would become the National Cancer Institute, now a division of the National Institutes of Health, testing three thousand compounds between 1935 and 1953. Only two of those compounds made it to clinical trials, and those were dropped because of unacceptable levels of toxicity.[16]

So, when Goodman and Gilman went to work in the 1940s, cancer treatment had not progressed much beyond surgery and in some cases radiation. Either or both *could* be very effective, but neither solved the problem of metastasis.

Goodman and Gilman used nitrogen mustard to shrink a tumor on a mouse that was larger than the mouse itself. The tumor returned, was shrunk again, and only on the third attempt did the tumor fail to respond. In 1942 they were able to keep a patient who could neither chew nor swallow alive for a month; for a short time, his tumors disappeared entirely. In 1943 sixty-seven patients around the country with advanced or terminal cancer were treated. Several died soon after the infusions began, as their veins shut down. The most noteworthy case, however, was that of a fifty-two-year-old man with leukemia and a white blood cell count of 293,000 per cubic milliliter. After nine months he appeared to be disease free and had normal blood counts.[17]

This one huge success among a multitude of lesser successes and abject failures was groundbreaking but, because of the terms of the military contract under which they worked, would have to remain top secret for many years.

After Germany fell, and two of Japan's major cities, Hiroshima and Nagasaki, were subjected to nuclear bombing, World War II effectively came to a close on August 15, 1945, when Japanese Emperor Hirohito announced surrender. The documents were subsequently signed on September 2 aboard the naval battleship USS *Missouri.* The results of the nitrogen-mustard experiments eventually would become public.

In a development that more or less paralleled the work of Goodman and Gilman, physician Sidney Farber, now called the father of chemotherapy, reported that the blood counts of children with leukemia who had been given an agent to block folic acid had returned to normal. Though Farber's article was cautiously worded, it generated considerable enthusiasm in the literature of the time and was instrumental in getting people to believe that effective chemotherapy was possible.[18]

The race for effective treatments for cancer was on. Between 1954 and 1964, one million mice were employed every year to test toxicity in 82,700 synthetic chemicals, 115,000 fermentation products, and 17,200 plant derivations.[19]

While enormous effort was made to find toxins[20] that killed cancer, efforts also were made in regard to administrating these toxins and later how to combine these agents for more effective treatment. The initial tests with mustard gas, as well as nitrogen mustard, eventually spawned several hundred chemotherapy treatments based on the poisoning principle. What these drugs do is attack cells in the process of division. Cancer cells divide very quickly, hence the effectiveness of the drugs. But the unpleasant side effects of chemo are the result of attacks on other cells that also divide rapidly.

Adult brain cells don't divide, and bone cells divide rarely, except in the event of injury. Chemotherapy doesn't attack these cells at all. At the other end of the spectrum are cells that do divide quickly, and chemotherapy does affect them. Hair-follicle cells divide every thirty to sixty minutes, so hair loss is usual. Cells in the stomach divide every two days, so nausea is common, though it usually can be effectively treated.[21] White blood cells divide every three days; platelets, which help form blood clots, every ten days; and red blood cells divide every three or four months. All blood cells are produced in the bone marrow; the side effects of this assault on the bone marrow and blood cells include fatigue and vulnerability to infection.

Why all the chemo sessions? An Alabama doctor named Howard Skipper came up with the fractional kill hypothesis, which states that a given percentage of cancer cells are killed with each chemotherapy session. Generally if a chemotherapy dosage can kill 99 percent of the existing cancer cells, it would take about six sessions to eradicate the cancer. Though the fractional kill hypothesis has been supported by animal studies and in the test tube, the exact mathematics is often disrupted by other factors, and it is usually impossible for oncologists to be certain the cancer is eradicated from the patient. For patients with peritoneal carcinomatosis, like Lisa, the presence of multiple cancers at once throws a monkey wrench into Skipper's hypothesis. There is, however, the remarkable story of a certain Dr. Min Chiu Li, who was able to achieve the very certainty that Skipper sought in a case of a rare placental cancer.

Doctor Min Chiu Li had graduated from medical school at Mukden University of China and in 1956 was subsequently working at the National Institutes of Health in Bethesda, Maryland. While he was on call one night, a woman was admitted with late-stage metastatic choriocarcinoma, which originates with the placental tissue. Li attempted to stabilize her, but she bled to death within three hours, apparently before his eyes. He decided that if he ever had a case like this again he would try one of Sidney Farber's antifolates, methotrexate. A few weeks later, a young woman named Ethel Longoria was admitted with the same condition. After four sessions, antifolates made the tumor disappear. Li was not satisfied. The choriocarcinoma cells that had made up the tumor secreted a protein called choriogonadotropin (CG or β-HCG), and it was still in the blood. In spite of the potential dangers of excess cytotoxicity, Li administered continuous doses until the CG level was zero. The woman was cured, but Li was eventually fired. His colleague, Doctor Emil Frierich, a heavyweight in oncology circles in his own right, found Li inconsolable in the wake of the firing. Li did all right, though, latching on with Memorial Sloan-Kettering, developing an effective chemotherapy program for metastatic testicular cancer, and sharing the prestigious Lasker Award for a major contribution to medicine in 1972—ironically with the man responsible for his firing, National Institutes of Health director Gordon Zubrod. In fairness to Doctor Zubrod, he apparently would have been willing to keep Li on if he agreed to stop using his regimen, but Li, not surprisingly, would not agree. Oncologist and writer Doctor Siddhartha Mukherjee has christened Li "the patron saint of renegades."[22]

Wouldn't it be great if other cancers responded to a similar treatment? The catch is that Doctor Li had success because CG is *only* present when placental cancer cells are present or when a woman is pregnant. Most tumor markers are found in a normal blood sample, and *elevated* levels of a tumor marker are an indication, but not proof, of cancer.

While recovering at home from her extensive operation, Lisa received several visits from Helen Szablya, a patient of Doctor Sardi's who took it upon herself to share her experiences of having gone through the process with newer patients who asked for her help.

Helen talked to Lisa about what she could expect to happen over the next year or so, including what to expect from chemotherapy. Helen had discontinued her chemotherapy sessions a bit early, as the sores she had developed in her mouth and the loss of sensation in her feet had proven too discomforting. Later Lisa brought these things up with Doctor Sardi, who told her to keep an open mind. The chemotherapy experience is different for each person, he said. Sardi proved to be right. Though the experience wasn't always pleasant, Lisa never did develop mouth sores or encounter neuropathy, and the neuropathy she had experienced as a result of the operation disappeared by about the fourteenth week. She also never completely lost her hair, though it did thin out considerably.

During his fellowship at Ohio State, Doctor Sardi had been happy working with Doctor Minton and his colleagues, and Minton had sounded Sardi out on becoming a partner there. Because he liked variety, Sardi found the position attractive. He could do clinical work, as his first love was working with patients, but he also could teach and do research. He had cobbled together $20,000 in grant money after he had arrived there, and he was proud of the initiative he had shown. When the grant was up, a senior administrator told him he would need to get a $500,000 grant from the National Institutes of Health to stay on. He did not think that would happen, so he began to apply to other institutions.

At the time his experience in submitting applications was very different from when South Baltimore had canceled its internship program. Then he had had only one offer in hand, from a New York hospital. He had gotten as far as being granted the chance to take a written exam and make a presentation at the prestigious Massachusetts General Hospital, but the competition there had been keen, and he was not accepted. Even Saint Agnes was not going to interview Sardi until his colleagues at South Baltimore called Doctor John Singer and urged him do so.

This time around it seemed everyone wanted him. According to Doctor Sardi, there were only nineteen surgical oncologists in the country at that time. He had six offers in hand, and in weighing them, he finally chose the Ochsner Clinic in New Orleans. They were offering an attractive ratio of clinical time to teaching and research, as well as the highest pay. Before he left, Ohio State contacted him to say that with or without the National Institutes of Health grant, he was welcome to stay, but Doctor Sardi had made a commitment, so he and his family moved to New Orleans.

It proved to be a good decision. He was impressed with the quality of the people around him, and he picked up a pair of Spirit of Caring Awards for his compassionate treatment of patients. He also taught himself laparoscopic surgery, adopting the surgeries he already knew well to the new technology, a bit like building a model ship inside a bottle. In 1992 he made a film for the American College of Surgeons about how to do a splenectomy, the removal of the spleen, using laparoscopic technology. He put the spleen in a zip-lock freezer bag he had sterilized, which drew a few chuckles when the film was shown. The makers of medical equipment, never to miss an opportunity, then designed a dedicated splenectomy bag, charging $300. Sardi later taught courses in laparoscopic surgery in Central America, South America, and Baltimore.

During Dr. Sardi's time at the Ochsner clinic, he began to follow the clinical publications of Doctor Paul Sugarbaker and was impressed with the results the doctor was generating. At the time, American medical orthodoxy, at least in patient consultations, often labeled Sugarbaker's work radical, or ignored it, or both. Sardi understood that the length of Sugarbaker's surgeries was building on the work of John Peter Minton and others, such as Doctor Owen Wangensteen of the University of Minnesota. The goal of completely removing all visible tumor from the peritoneum during a single surgery was unique but, to Sardi's mind, probably not impossible. He wanted to learn more.

Doctor Sardi invited Doctor Sugarbaker to give a presentation at the Ochsner Clinic and, to help make Sugarbaker's stay in New Orleans more relaxed, invited him to stay with the Sardi family. In this way the two men could just chat. Sardi was so impressed with Sugarbaker's conversation and presentation that when he returned to Baltimore in 1994 he built his own perfusion pump with some parts purchased at Radio Shack and elsewhere and, with guidance from Sugarbaker, initiated a HIPEC program. The pump he built for about $400 back in the day can cost up to $250,000 now, with the stipulation that $3,000 in new tubing be used for each operation.

Back at Saint Agnes Hospital, Doctor John Singer put together a very attractive package to bring back Doctor Sardi, who then told his boss at the Ochsner Clinic, Doctor Larry Hollier, that he wanted to return to Saint Agnes.

Doctor Hollier had received his Bachelor of Science degree from Louisiana State University in Baton Rouge and his medical degree at the Louisiana State University Medical School in New Orleans. After a circuitous route, he found himself at the Ochsner Clinic, about five miles from the medical school. In addition to his administrative skills, he had many clinical interests, and although he was primarily a heart specialist, his additional expertise in eye surgery, more formally known as ophthalmic surgery or ocular surgery, would make him an especially attractive candidate to be in charge of hiring and training at a brand-new for-profit hospital. If Sardi were planning on leaving Ochsner anyway, Sardi, who himself had a full toolbox of surgical technique and specialties, might prove a trusted lieutenant.

A company, Health Care International, Ltd., was planning on building three hospitals, one in Scotland, one in Singapore, and one in Brazil to accommodate patients who had the means to bypass some of the socialist health-care systems that then had backlogs. In England at the time, for example, cardiac patients had to wait up to two years to undergo surgery, and many died while waiting.

As it was with the fictitious character of John Hammond in Michael Chrichton's *Jurassic Park*, Health Care International and its investors spared no expense. A group of New England architects created a cluster of buildings made of brick, concrete, and glass. There was an MRI in the operating room. All the equipment was state-of-the-art. Next door was the 168-room four-star Beardmore Hotel and Conference Center. The hospital was an eight-mile drive from the Glasgow International Airport. Construction of the hospital cost £180 million, which would have been about $400 million in American dollars.

Such a hospital would need a crackerjack staff. Doctor Hollier lobbied Doctor Sardi to join him, and when Sardi agreed, he was one of fifteen doctors recruited from the United States, with several more recruited in Europe. Dr. Sardi was the youngest in the group and the first to arrive.

For the first nine months, the hospital was open to medical staff but not patients. During this time Doctor Sardi flew to various European cities, talking up the hospital, but he spent most of his time training doctors, nurses, and staff and setting up logistics.

The procedures of most hospitals have evolved over time. Mercy Hospital in Baltimore, as mentioned, opened as a teaching hospital where new doctors could learn their trade by treating the poor who could not afford more experienced doctors. It took more than a century for it to be considered a top hospital in the United States.

In 1993, however, everything had to be put in place at the hospital in Scotland over months, not years or even decades. All groups within a hospital interact with other groups, and communication channels needed to be established.

The medical teams started at eight or later in the morning and, with no patients, knocked off around four. The relatively short hours were partly a matter of Scottish custom and partly necessitated by the public transportation system.

When the hospital opened its doors, patients trickled in, and enrollment never reached expectations. The planned hospitals in Singapore and Brazil were never built. In 2002 the hospital was sold to the United Kingdom; the name was changed to the Golden Jubilee National Hospital; and it has since served the public. Several cutting-edge technologies have emerged at the hospital, most notably the use of computer-navigation surgery in joint replacement.

The hospital has become a success story after all, and Health Care International, Ltd., is still in business, though it looks like they've been pared down to their core strength, providing health-care coverage. Still, a hospital that had cost £180 million to build was sold for a mere £37.5 million. What went wrong?

The original name, the National Waiting Times Centre, would be puzzling to many outside of England, and marketing also may have been a problem. Clyde Bank, outside Glasgow, was a six-hour drive from London.

Doctor Sardi, when asked what he might do if given a chance to go back in history to fix what happened, observed that the hospital probably should have been built twenty years earlier. Another possibility is that the hospital might have done better with a few key specialties, adding buildings, doctors, and staff as its reputation grew. Then again that would have been a different concept altogether.

Doctor Sardi left after the hospital had been open for three months. He was the first to arrive, the second to leave. A local newspaper article mentioned that there weren't enough patients there for him, and he may even have expressed surprise or disappointment at this lack of patients at some point, but that was only part of the reason he left.

His wife was miserable, as were several of the wives of the imported medical professionals. Though the Scottish people were hospitable, his wife was unhappy living in a place that had two seasons, winter and June, as Doctor Sardi later quipped.

He went back to Saint Agnes mostly to keep his wife happy and was stunned, twelve years later, when she told him she was leaving for good. By then their two daughters were grown, and his wife was absorbed with her interior design business. Indulging in a bit of introspective writing helped Sardi get through those difficult times, and afterward he felt he probably would marry again but, consistent with his incurably passionate outlook, only if he were to fall in love.

Lisa postponed her first regular chemotherapy session until after Thanksgiving. She wanted to ensure that her blood count was sufficient for us to allow friends and family over.

This was the first year since we had moved to our row home nineteen years previously that Thanksgiving wasn't held in the dining room. The dining room had become Lisa's office, and the dining-room table had been pushed up against the buffet. Above the doorways were Beatrix Potter plates. In one corner a yellowed article had been framed—something Lisa had written years before for *The Baltimore Sun*.

The dining-room table was now in the middle of the living room, which was graced with plants and Lisa's original art and had just enough room for people to get in and out of their seats comfortably. Among our guests were Doctor Marcy Roenneberg and her daughter, who had accompanied her mother on her trips to Niger and Bangladesh. Her daughter was now a senior in college.

I was explaining to my sister Marie, who was visiting from Buffalo, that although Marcy was an occasional Thanksgiving guest, this year was *extra* special because Marcy had been instrumental in getting us to Doctor Sardi. As I explained this, I cut through the crisp, golden brown skin of the turkey, placed a portion on a porcelain plate, and passed the plate to Marcy.

The next day Lisa looked out the living-room window in the early afternoon. All but a few stubborn leaves had fallen from the trees, and Danny and I were gathering those that had been raked into piles..

Chemo would begin in a few days.

Five

Pooh, promise you won't forget about me, ever. Not even when I'm a hundred.--from A.A. Milne's The House on Pooh Corner

While Doctor Sardi and Doctor Gushchin anchor one side of the fourth floor of the Weinberg Center, Doctor Payotis (Peter) Ledakis anchors the other. Ledakis is from Athens, Greece, and graduated from the University of Athens Medical School. He served his residency at the Albert Einstein Medical Center in Philadelphia, Pennsylvania, founded in the 1860s as the Jewish Hospital for the Aged, Infirmed and Destitute, though the hospital provided care for the suffering poor of all religions. There Ledakis met his wife, Carol Phillips, the daughter of two National Institutes of Health researchers; she eventually would become a doctor of obstetrics and gynecology.

Doctor Ledakis served a fellowship at the National Cancer Institute and the National Blood Institute, a division of NIH, in oncology and hematology. He and his wife then practiced medicine in Nebraska, where he also served as an associate professor. There he earned a third certification as a diplomat in hematology to go along with his certifications in oncology and internal medicine.

His decision to join the Mercy team in Baltimore was a bit of a homecoming for his wife, as she could work part-time and let her mother help with the kids, at least when her mother wasn't traveling to Mongolia, Italy, or Antarctica.

Doctor Ledakis, who carries a professorial air about him, recently served as a mentor for engineering students who developed a fiber-optic bone-marrow biopsy needle, designed to be more accurate than a needle that had no light source. He was also one of the doctors featured in the 2012 article "My Doctor Saved My Life!" His patient, who had received a timely second opinion from him, also noted his compassionate manner. In the article, Ledakis responded, "Some doctors feel more effective if they remain detached, but I think it's better if you try to communicate and connect. We all suffer in different ways."[1]

Doctor Ledakis is well aware that oncologists are moving to therapies that specifically target cancer cells, or molecules expressed on cancer cells, and one of the rapidly growing fields is immunology, in which doctors are attempting to harness the body's own immune system to recognize cancer.

Can you train white blood cells to do this? This possibility was more or less established in the 1800s, though continued progress in this direction was apparently eclipsed by the later promise of radiation therapy, as well as the skepticism of many physicians at that time.

In the 1800s? After all, the concept of tumorigenesis, the production or formation of a tumor, had not even been articulated, and although the pronounced differences in white blood types could be seen under a microscope, the interaction among them was poorly understood. The concept was established empirically through observation and experiment, but proof of principle can be teased out.

After one of his patients, Elizabeth Dashielle, died of bone cancer, a bone surgeon named William Coley began to research similar cases. He found the records of a certain Fred Stein, whose bone tumor had disappeared after he contracted an erysipelas infection, which would now be known as Streptococcus pyogenes. He also found that medical pioneers Louis Pasteur, Emil von Behring, and Robert Koch—the same Robert Koch we met in the last chapter and who originally defined the cause of infectious diseases—had made the same observation. Unknown to Coley at the time, Russian physician and writer Anton Chekhov also had recorded the same observation.

In 1891 Doctor Coley intentionally infected a certain Mr. Zola, who was suffering from tonsil and throat cancer, with Streptococcus pyogenes; his condition improved dramatically, and he went on to live another eight and a half years. Coley published his findings.[2]

By January 1893 Doctor Coley had produced a toxin—also referred to at the time as a vaccine and referred to today as Coley's fluid—and injected the toxin into the massive abdominal cancer of John Ficken, a sixteen-year-old boy. The injections continued every few days, with enough toxin to produce a fever but not the disease itself. By August the tumor was almost imperceptible. Having achieved several successes, in 1893 he published the results of his treatment of nine other patients as well.[3] John Ficken died of a heart attack twenty-six years later, at age forty-two.

There is no claim here that Doctor Coley set out to train white blood cells to attack cancer. There is probably even a plausible explanation out there somewhere that he could accomplish what he did without reorienting the white blood cells at all.

Doctor Coley was doing what doctors generally try to do when treating patients before all the details of the science have been worked out step by step. He made an observation, found that the observation had been confirmed by others in the field, stumbled upon a possible remedy, and then recorded his results. Many doctors at the time didn't trust his findings, and a few years later, radiation was discovered and was believed to be the miracle cure for cancer, putting Coley's discoveries on the back burner. In many ways radiation did work quite well; today, tumors that have not metastasized often can be incinerated without a surgeon ever cutting into the body. Ironically, though, radiation never has been as effective against metastasis as Coley's toxin was, assuming, of course, that Coley hadn't fudged his results.[4]

It's possible that chemotherapy has evolved to the point where it is now safer than Coley's toxins. After all, of the estimated 700 million individuals naturally infected by Streptococcus pyogenes annually, an estimated 260,000 of them die, but if the science behind why these toxins worked could be harnessed safely, a promising door to cancer therapy would be reopened.

Doctor Coley's fluid is still used in some places today. In Germany, for example, a doctor can use the toxin if he mixes a batch himself. The chief drawback, however, other than the fact that it's out of vogue, is that inconsistencies in its manufacture likely will keep regulatory bodies, including the FDA, from approving it.

Practical experience keeps many laypeople from intuitively understanding how diversified white blood cells really are. Blood is blood. It's *red*. Historical medical texts often mention suppuration, or the forming of pus, but in the days before microscopes, we weren't much beyond Hippocrates's four humors of black bile, yellow bile, blood, and phlegm, the last of which could have been construed as white blood cells, especially if one is observing blood separating into layers.[5]

Under a microscope, red blood cells all look alike and all do the same thing—carry nutrients and oxygen to all parts of the body and carry away waste. Platelets look alike, and all of them help stop leaks. But white blood cells look very different, and although they all more or less subscribe to the same mission statement, to bounce the riffraff from the premises, they really don't all do the same thing. It might be easier to view white blood cells as an army filled with warriors of different ranks and abilities, avenger cells, guardian cells, bodyguard cells, informer cells, and so on.

The three "phils"— neutrophils, eosinophils, and basophils—make up a tad less than two-thirds of the white blood cells, and as a simplification, they target the usual suspects: bacteria, fungi, and parasites. The remaining white blood cells are made up of the two "cytes," lymphocytes and monocytes, each of which has candidates to be recruited in the fight against cancer. Most chemotherapy carpet-bombs the countryside, potentially creating unacceptable collateral damage. For the cancers that chemo can treat at all, it is usually the best we have right now. But if the "cytes" could be safely recruited and properly trained—no easy task—they would be like stealth assassins, surreptitiously combing the countryside, taking out the cancer cells with little collateral damage.

Why can't these white blood cells take out the cancer anyway? As mentioned in chapter one, cancer cells evolve from our own cells and are often not recognized as foreign, however dangerous they may become.

Among the lymphocyte candidates are B cells, T cells, and NK, or natural killer cells. Helping to activate them are the monocytes, macrophages, and dendritic cells. Though candidates among white blood cells to recruit in the fight against cancer abound, training the dendritic cells in particular is one of the most promising therapies.

Dendritic cells, which make up less than 1 percent of all white blood cells, are found in most tissues of the body. They travel from the thymus gland to the skin, heart, kidneys, bloodstream, etc., and if not needed, they can stay there for the life of the organism. If they are needed to bounce the riffraff, they take the offender to the lymph nodes, where both the offender and dendritic cell die, with the old post taken up by a new dendritic cell. In the 1980s, Doctor Edgar Engleman of Stanford University's School of Medicine isolated white blood cells from blood samples then further isolated the dendritic cells, exposed them to cancer, and reintroduced the dendritic cells to the body, with successful results. The chief drawback to this therapy is apparently that a process that cost $500 or $600 in the 1980s would cost at least $30,000 today because of FDA regulation to ensure purity. Nonetheless the therapy continues to evolve.

Of the movement from toxins to targeted therapy, oncologist and writer Doctor Siddhartha Mukherjee notes:

The tools that we will use to battle cancer in the future will doubtless alter so dramatically in fifty years that the geography of cancer prevention and therapy might be unrecognizable. Future physicians may laugh at our mixing of primitive cocktails of poisons to kill the most elemental and magisterial disease known to our species.[6]

For Doctor Ledakis, a consummate problem solver, Lisa's case presented less certainty than most cases. A doctor's best friend is evidence-based medicine, therapies proven to work in clinical studies. For many cancers of the peritoneum, such as colon cancer or ovarian cancer, there was ample literature on which regimens worked well—not necessarily what was *ultimately* the best, but what was the best *so far,* what doctors refer to as the current standard of practice. All cases that included peritoneal carcimomatosis, however, were heterogenous in nature, involving a variety of tumors. In cases of colon cancer with peritoneal seeding, or of ovarian cancer with peritoneal seeding, there was less literature and therefore less certainty, but one could design a chemotherapy regimen based on colon cancer that had metastasized elsewhere or ovarian cancer that had metastasized elsewhere. In short, at least there was a logical place to start.

As mentioned, Lisa had had primary peritoneal carcinomatosis. There was sufficient literature on what had been tried before, but in the absence of clinical trials, there was nothing really on what was proven to work. More so than in many cases, Doctor Ledakis would need to interpret the blood samples, track the cancer markers over time, and be ready to tweak the regimen.

There was a further complication, a sort of adjunct to Skipper's cell kill hypothesis, that a constant fraction of the cancer cells are killed with each chemotherapeutic dose, necessitating many sessions. Even with what the surgeons call complete cytoreduction, the volume of tumor in peritoneal carcinomatosis can be large enough that drug-resistant cells will remain. As mentioned, cancer cells tend to divide quickly, and each new generation of cancer cells harbors mutated cells. According to the Goldie-Coldman model,[7] with a large enough initial volume, the existence of drug-resistant cancer is not probable, it is *certain*, which at the very least necessitates a multiple-drug regimen. The ghost of Howard Skipper would approve; at a time when NIH researchers were stuck on the protocol of testing one drug at a time, Skipper was sending word from Alabama that multiple-drug cocktails were working better on his mice than single agents. In the 1970s one rare cancer, Burkitt's lymphoma, was successfully treated with a seven-drug cocktail, though a better regimen is still being sought, and an eight-drug cocktail was suggested for Hodgkin's disease.[8]

Doctor Ledakis expected that even after chemotherapy and the subsequent maintenance, Lisa's cancer would return. When it did, he would start anew on the problem at hand and find the words to give her some reassurance.

Lisa's chemotherapy began on her third visit to Doctor Ledakis, as iron had been administered during the first two visits to help get her red blood cell count up.

On that third visit, after her IV was inserted, she passed out ever so briefly. At the time the attending nurse thought the chemotherapy had not started, but playing it safe, Doctor Ledakis scheduled another session for the following Tuesday, and not in the Weinberg Center but on the fifteenth floor of the Bunting Center, where Lisa had endured her long recovery.

Coincidentally, Lisa and I already had arranged to have sandwich wraps and potato salad delivered to the fifteenth floor, as well as the intensive care unit, as a thank-you for all the kindnesses afforded her. The latter gesture provided more foreshadowing than we would have liked.

On the fifteenth floor, Lisa passed out, came to, passed out again, and stopped breathing. Twenty or more people swarmed the room as well as the corridor outside the room. The clergy, fine people all, sequestered me to one corner of the hospital or another, and I found a subject of common interest with a beneficent priest, Father James Joyce, the topic of interest being the life and works of the Trappist monk Thomas Merton, whose writings had influence my everyday conduct probably more than any other writer. I had had the chance to look over Merton's unpublished diary, kept in a cooled vault in the library of my alma mater, Saint Bonaventure University, and the priest's willingness to engage me in conversation calmed my frayed nerves considerably. Lisa, meanwhile, was whisked away to the intensive care unit, where she stayed overnight.

When Marcy told Lisa if she would do everything Doctor Sardi recommended she would go on to see our son do great things, Marcy had been on speakerphone. Marcy sounded certain, and I latched on to that certainty. As a result, Lisa had experienced countless terrors while I had not. On that Tuesday on the fifteenth floor, I was forced to go through just once what my wife had gone through many times.

A cell phone of hers again disappeared. When she recovered her old phone number, she was subjected to fielding calls for weeks afterward, calls for Derrell, whoever and wherever he may have been.

Doctor Ledakis identified one of the chemotherapeutic agents as the likely culprit and removed it from the regimen. Playing it doubly safe, he scheduled Lisa's next chemotherapy session in the intensive care unit. The attending nurse told Lisa she never had administered chemo in the ICU, though Lisa was not entirely enamored with the thought that she might now be a *very* minor historical personage. The session was uneventful, as were all her subsequent sessions.

Lisa's employer had a program that allowed employees to donate some of their leave time to others who needed it, so she was able to recuperate for about five months. Even after five months, however, she probably wasn't completely herself, but the alternative, applying for disability, was unattractive to her.

Her return was bittersweet. Her closest colleagues were glad to have her back, of course, but others did not recognize her. She had left with medium-length black hair and returned with short, thinned-out, salt-and-pepper hair. She also had lost seventy pounds.

It was more than not being recognized. She sometimes felt like a character in a Tennessee Williams play, on the periphery of things rather than in the center. She felt lower in the pecking order. There wasn't necessarily anything insidious about this, as some people probably never expected to see her again.

She also probably had become oversensitive to what a big fuss others made about every little thing. Her perspective had changed, but she wouldn't call this new perspective any sort of enlightenment, as she would not necessarily wish her new perspective on those who hadn't been through something similar. If anything she sometimes envied the way others *could* make a fuss about every little thing.

Her giving up alcohol, not because her HIPEC treatment necessitated it, but because of her cirrhosis, also probably exacerbated her sense of being on the periphery. She would be seeing less of her colleagues after hours.

In spring 2012, on one of his trips back to Colombia, Doctor Armando Sardi tied the knot with his sweetheart, Mavalynne. In spring 2010, one of his sisters-in-law had insisted he take her out on a low-key date at a pizzeria, just to chat. Sardi had remembered Mavalynne, but as they had both been married to someone else at the time, he barely had noticed her before.

On that night in 2010, however, he was very taken with her. He quips that he had wanted to feel butterflies again, but on that night felt birds. On her part, she had admired the fact that a man of his standing would come back to Colombia year after year to help the poor. In 2012 they had a relatively small wedding at a club, with dinner and dancing afterward. Though divorced Catholics cannot marry in a church, the newlyweds were nonetheless graced with a blessing, by one of Armando Sardi's brothers, who was a priest.

In summer 2012, in a ceremony held in Mexico City, Doctor Jesus Esquivel, whom we met briefly in chapter one, was inducted into the Mexican Academy of Surgery, an august body of surgeons from around the world that is kept at a constant membership of four hundred. For each member that passes away, a new member is chosen. Almost certainly Esquivel's many trips back to Mexico, sometimes with Doctor Sugarbaker, to teach HIPEC technique to local surgeons, contributed to his being selected.

Doctor Esquivel has now traded in one of his slides, the one reminding us of the gravitational challenge of jumping from airplanes, for another, one that quotes Nobel Prize-winning Max Planck—"A new scientific truth does not triumph by winning its opponents and making them see the light, but rather because its opponents eventually die and a new generation grows up that is familiar with it."

Doctor Vadim Gushchin, who joined the Mercy team in 2006, graduated from the Russian State University in 1993 after six years then began his surgical residency there. He finished his residency at Washington Hospital Center in 2004, working with Doctor Paul Sugarbaker and winning two awards for surgical excellence and another for academic excellence. He also has received surgical oncology training in Roswell Park, Buffalo, and has been trained in advanced pancreatic surgery in Germany and advanced gastric surgery in Japan. Of the latter he has said that the West is skeptical of the impressive clinical results coming out of Japan; the problem is that American and Western surgeons believe they are performing the same surgery, but they are not.

Doctor Gushchin's English is very good, and he's adept at making contributions to the language. Surgeons are operators, and HIPEC coordinators, navigators, for example, as in "How does one become a good operator?" and "I can't diminish the role of the good navigator in this case."

When Doctor Gushchin first stepped into Doctor Paul Sugarbaker's operating room during a cytoreduction surgery, his first reaction was to leave and never come back. It did not seem this could *possibly* be the correct treatment option. He eventually was won over, though, and at one point helped set up a HIPEC facility in Siberia. He built his own perfusion pump, which as of 2013 was still in use, in spite of his imploring them to spring for an upgrade.

Doctor Gushchin had made the rounds of the fifteenth floor during Lisa's stay there and had become acquainted with her. Now Lisa was back to hear Doctor Sardi interpret the results of her first six-month CT scan, an anxiety-filled moment. In addition Sardi was temporarily out of the office, so Lisa had time to convince herself of the worst, if that was what she was wont to do. If Gushchin were guessing at how he could alleviate some of Lisa's anxiety, he guessed right.

"So," he said jokingly, poking his head through the doorway, "why exactly are you here again?!"

By August 2012 Lisa had finished her regular chemotherapy regimen as well as three of six maintenance appointments. Maintenance was chemo light, sort of, with two drugs in the regimen rather than three and visits scheduled every four weeks rather than every three. The concept behind maintenance has been around for a while; it would be designed, in Lisa's case, to hinder a recurrence of her cancer. It is increasingly recommended by oncologists, partly because the side effects of the various chemotherapy regimens have become more tolerable.

Two events would be coming up—the *Heat It to Beat It Walk* that Doctor Sardi's patients had started and Lisa's second six-month CT scan. She was not looking forward to the CT scan at all, a condition known to cancer survivors as "scanxiety." As she told this to the nurse administering her fourth maintenance dosage, the nurse told her that she herself had had cancer eight years ago and that she was still getting regularly scheduled CT scans. The nurse still found the experience frightening. Then, after a long silence, the nurse added, almost with a shade of embarrassment, "My husband tells me I just have to get over it."

As though it were just that simple.

The 2012 *Heat It to Beat It* walk began and ended at Rash Field, at the south end of Baltimore's Inner Harbor. Rash Field hosts competitive and pickup volleyball on seven courts built on one thousand or so tons of sand. Moving toward the water's edge, one can get a view of the Inner Harbor, the sea vessels docked there, the water taxis, and the colorful paddle boats, many of which are made to resemble sea dragons. It was a pleasant, sunny day.

A disc jockey was set up beneath the pavilion to provide dance music for the young and young at heart after the walk. On one side a hospitality tent staffed by volunteers handled the registration and handed out T-shirts. On the other side, fruit, water, bagels, and chewy bars were provided, and just beyond that, two pillars of red and orange balloons marked both the beginning and the end of the walk.

Everyone signing up for the event was eligible for the annual T-shirt, and this year the main color was that of sockeye salmon. Many of the teams had provided their own shirts or sweatshirts, the most noticeable of them being Nancy's Red Hot Crab Attackers. They also had come with matching headgear—cross-eyed, cartoonish crabs whose protruding claws wiggled as the teammates walked.

Though the initial goal had been to raise $100,000, more than eight hundred people showed up and raised more than $140,000.

Doctor Sardi had remarked that he always liked looking out over the crowd. In 2010 a woman called him to say she was coming to the walk; she had undergone HIPEC surgery performed by one of the doctors Sardi had trained. She also said she was Len Cynkar's wife.

That brought back memories for Doctor Sardi. Len Cynkar was an athlete who held seven records at Mosinee High School, unbroken even after forty years. One of those records, in track and field, he shared with Armando Sardi. The young Sardi was a good athlete in his own right, but his telling of the story was a bit reminiscent of an anecdote that NBA player and coach Al Attles was fond of telling, of the crisp night in Hershey, Pennsylvania, before four thousand plus spectators, when Wilt Chamberlain and he had combined for 117 points.

Doctor Sardi, wearing the salmon-colored shirt, blue jeans, and a white baseball cap, stood just in front of the pavilion and took the microphone. He stressed how much of his work was really a team effort, calling his colleagues at Mercy the most dedicated he ever had worked with. A dozen or more nurses from the hospital cheered him on. Later he pointed out family members who had come: his daughters, his son-in-law, his grandchildren, his wife, and his mother. He choked up explaining to them that all the times he had come home late because of his work, he was always thinking of them. He collected himself, and to sympathetic laughter, he admitted, "I get emotional and cry sometimes, but I'm glad that I can." He acknowledged the many groups who had participated, talked about what had been accomplished in the previous year, and finished by quoting Winston Churchill—"Never, never, *never* give up!"

After Doctor Gushchin spoke very briefly, the crowd moved toward the starting area.

A few people, service personnel who worked in the Inner Harbor, looked earnestly out at the crowd of migrating salmon. Maybe some members of the crowd would come back to grace their establishments when this walk was over, as business had not been good for years. Surely *some* of them would come back.

A friend of Lisa's, Marianne, had put together a team on Lisa's behalf. The previous year they had walked around the harbor while she was recuperating in a hospital bed. This year Lisa and I were joining them, and Lisa got everyone's attention by quoting a line from the television show *Glee*, something about being told she didn't have to give a speech, but she was giving one anyway. She thanked her team from the bottom of her heart, saying she couldn't have made it through without them. She ending her short speech choking on her words. "I just know how much love is out there. It makes life worth living. That's all there is, and that's all I'm going to say."

It was a little bit awkward, but only a little. They had not done *that* much, visiting her a few times and marching around the Inner Harbor, but it was a good thing that what they had done had meant so much. Lisa did not have what they actually had done in mind as much as the thought that they would be awaiting her return from the rabbit hole, that during those nights when the beaches of Thailand would float by on the screen, she could think of all the people who would be glad to see her again, if she could only make it through. They understood what she meant.

Then they too merged into the crowd, the few among the many, taking in the pleasant, sunny September day until they arrived back to where they started, then going out together for brunch, all the while discussing—what else?—all the latest!

Twenty minutes or so into the walk, Lisa was chatting with one of her teammates, Doug, who had brought her some cheery Mylar balloons the night before her surgery more than a year before. He had very recently lost a brother to suicide after a protracted battle with addictive drugs. Doug recalled the last conversation he had had with his brother and said he realized at the time that he finally could become friends with him again, finally, *finally*, after all those years of his brother telling him only what he thought Doug wanted to hear and their drifting further and further apart. It turned out there would be no time for a genuine and extended reconciliation, but it is common for people, after the loss of a loved one, or a former loved one, to revisit all the little things they might have done differently.

Maybe it's the same for many of us—to hope that in life the fond memories somehow eclipse the regrets.

Lisa filled a gap in the conversation by changing the subject. "Would you believe this whole thing was started by Doctor Sardi's *patients*?"

"That's an interesting position to be in," said Doug. "He's already a highly regarded doctor, and then he's liked by all these people..."

"*Loved!*" someone interjected.

Doug hesitated, taking it all in.

It would be a bit much if all these people were here *just* for Doctor Sardi, who, like anyone else, had experienced both success and disappointment. One *could* believe, however, that

Armando Sardi represented something greater than himself and that the perpetual compassion and optimism and happiness that emanated from his faith were at least a little bit contagious.

There is no cure for many cancers. There may never be. There are not enough doctors for the children of South America or for the untouchables of Africa. It is sometimes difficult for decent people to accept how unfair life can be for so many others who deserve better. Yet for one courageous and fortunate woman, faced with the prospect that there would be few tomorrows, healed, at least so far, beneath the hands of a gifted surgeon, the chance to see her most precious dreams fulfilled had come to pass.

Acknowledgments

Lisa and I would like to thank Dr. Armando Sardi and his staff: Nick Athas, PA-C; Dr. Vadim Gushchin; Sara Keihl; Stephanie Lackey, PA-C; Dr. Suven Shankar; and practice manager Jennifer Francis. We also would like to welcome newcomer Dr. Kurtis A. Campbell.

Thanks to Mercy Hospital's Dr. Payotis (Peter) Ledakis; Dr. Robert Lydell; Dr. Paul Tuluvath; Harriet Pilert, RN; and Sabina Kang, PA-C.

Thanks to others who took the time to talk to me: Dr. John Singer; Dr. Marcella Roenneberg; Carole Langrall; Marie Henderson, RSM, Maria Muscovin; and several others in the field of oncology who were helpful, encouraging, or both. Any oversimplifications or mistakes are my fault.

Thanks to Ilse Sugarbaker for helping me locate difficult-to-find material.

Thanks to the staff at CreateSpace, including Travis Craine, Kristen, Callie, Josh and especially Angela.

In addition to other sources mentioned in the endnotes, I would like to point out that the material at hipectreatment. com was extremely helpful, as was material put out by the PMP Foundation. Siddhartha Mukherjee's *The Emperor of All Maladies: A Biography of Cancer* was especially valuable. Helpful and concise are Judith McKay and Tamera Schacher's *The Chemotherapy Survival Guide,* third edition, which should answer any patient's practical questions about chemotherapy, and Tomasz M. Beer and Larry W. Axmaker's *Cancer Clinical Trials*, which should answer any patient's practical questions about clinical trials.

Though I did only a small amount of primary research at the site, Wikipedia proved to be extremely valuable as a fact-checker, as a resource for more detail, and as a resource to locate older or even original sources.

Armando Sardi, MD, FACS
Curriculum Vitae

(As of October, 2013)

DEGREES
M.D. Universidad del Valle
Cali, Colombia - S.A.
1973-1980

POST GRADUATE TRAINING
Hospital Santander
San Andres Island, Colombia - S.A.
1980-1981 Rural Service*

* Required by the Colombian Ministry of Education and Health
for all medical graduates of Colombia.

INTERNSHIP
Universidad del Valle
Cali, Colombia - S.A.
1979-1980 Rotating Internship

South Baltimore General Hospital
Baltimore, MD, U.S.A
1981-1982 Surgical Intern

RESIDENCY
South Baltimore General Hospital
Baltimore, Maryland - U.S.A.
1982-1983 Surgical Resident

Saint Agnes Hospital
Baltimore, Maryland - U.S.A.
1983-1985 Surgical Resident

Saint Agnes Hospital
Baltimore, Maryland - U.S.A.
1985-1986 Surgical Oncology Fellow & Surgical Chief Resident

FELLOWSHIP
Ohio State University Hospital
Division of Surgical Oncology
Columbus, Ohio - U.S.A.
1986-1988

American Cancer Society
Clinical Fellowship Grant
1987-1988

LICENSURE
State of Maryland
State of Ohio
State of Louisiana
United Kingdom

CERTIFICATIONS
American Board of Surgery
NIH certified on the Protection of Human Research Subjects
(12/2000)

HONORS AND AWARDS
- Full scholarship for occupying first place (1/95) in medical school. March 1974 through February 1975.
- Full scholarship for attaining/receiving first place (1/92) in medical school. April 1975 through March 1976.
- Cianos Award - Saint Agnes Hospital. June 1984, (awarded to the surgical resident who has demonstrated more extensive knowledge in basic sciences).
- Cianos Award - Saint Agnes Hospital. June 1986, (awarded to the surgical resident who has demonstrated more extensive knowledge in basic sciences).
- First place winner, Ohio Chapter American College of Surgeons Resident Essay Contest, "Localization of tumor labeled with antibody 'cocktail' by hand-held gamma probe", 1988.

- Second place winner, Ohio Chapter of the American College of Surgeons Resident Essay Contest, "The use of a hand-held gamma detector improves the safety of isolated limb perfusion", 1988.
- "The Spirit of Caring" Award, Ochsner Clinic, New Orleans, LA, 1991-1993.
- Teacher of the Year and Outstanding Attending in General Surgery, 1996-97 by the Surgical House staff at St. Agnes Hospital.
- "Hands Humanitarian Award", by the Hands Across America
  Organization in recognition of his voluntary treatment for children in need throughout America, Baltimore, Maryland. November 30, 2001.
- Governor's Citation of the State of Maryland for the successful mission in Hands Across America, Inc. November 30, 2001.
- Founder's Award for the year 2003. This physician of the year award is given to the physician that has demonstrated performance as an exemplary physician during his years of service at St. Agnes HealthCare.
- The Daily Record, Healthcare Heroes Award for "Advancements in Healthcare." Baltimore, Maryland. March 28, 2007.
- "Premio Colombia Exterior A La Excelecia 2007." This award was presented for excellence in science. Broadway, NY. May 11, 2007.
- "Hispanic Hero" at the 3rd Annual Maryland Hispanic Youth Symposium. Baltimore, Maryland. July 19, 2007.

- "Gold Star Caregiver Award." Presented by The Sisters of Mercy in recognition of Gold Star Care performance and patient compliments. September 4, 2007.
- "Visitante Ilustre De Santiago De Cali." Presented by the Mayor of City of Cali, Colombia. February 26, 2008.
- Gobernador Citation Valle Del Cauca – Colombia for the contribution to improve the quality of life of the poorest and more vulnerable people. February 26, 2008.
- "La Medalla Santiago de Cali en el Grado Cruz de Oro." Presented by Concejo Municipal of City of Cali, Colombia. February 29, 2008.
- "Hispanic Hero Award for Excellence as a Medical/Social Entrepreneur." Presented by USHYEE. Baltimore, MD. June 5, 2008.
- Honored by Baltimore Magazine as "Top Doc." Baltimore, MD November 2009
- "Gold Star Teamwork Award." Presented by The Sisters of Mercy in recognition of Gold Star performance. December 2009
- Honored by Baltimore Magazine as "Top Doc." Baltimore, MD November 2011
- Honored by Baltimore Magazine as "Top Doc." Baltimore, MD November 2012
- Honored by Fusionarte as one of "100 Colombianos" who represent the talent, creativity and perseverance of Colombia. Bogota, Colombia December 2012

SPECIAL EXAMINATIONS
1. ECFMG - January 21, 1981

2. FLEX - State of Maryland, June 1982
3. American Board of Surgery

MEDICAL ASSOCIATIONS
1. American College of Surgeons
2. Society of Surgical Oncology
3. American Society of Clinical Oncology
4. The Society for Surgery of the Alimentary Tract
5. Medical and Chirurgical Faculty of Maryland
6. Southeastern Surgical Association
7. American Medical Association
8. Association of the Alumni of the "Division de Salud of the Universidad del Valle
9. National Cancer Institute - Clinical Investigator

APPOINTMENTS
- Staff Surgical Oncology - General Surgery, Alton Ochsner Medical Foundation. July 1, 1988 through August 31, 1993.
- Clinical Assistant Professor of Surgery, Tulane University Medical Center. 1988 -1993
- Medical Director, Surgical Technology Program, Ochsner School of Allied Health Sciences. 1990 -1993.
- Louisiana District #1 Committee on Applicants of the American College of Surgeons. 1991 - 1993.
- Founding Chief of the Division of Surgical Oncology, Health Care International (Scotland) Ltd. September 1, 1993 - August 12, 1994.
- Co-Director of Oncology Program, Health Care International (Scotland) Ltd. Sept. 1, 1993 - Aug. 12, 1994

- Member of Editorial board of the Maryland Medical Journal (MMJ), 1996-1997.
- Member of the membership committee of the Society of Head and Neck Surgeons - 1997 – 1998
- Member of Editorial Board of Clinical Researcher, June 2000 to July 2003
- Chief of Surgical Oncology, Saint Agnes HealthCare. August 15, 1994 – January 31, 2006
- Founding Medical Director, Clinical Research Center, St. Agnes HealthCare, January 1998 – January 31, 2006
- Faculty and Preceptor for Ethicon Endosurgery Institute. For the education and development of physicians in the area of minimally invasive techniques. – 2003 – present.
- Member of the Scientific Council of Colombia Médica-Universidad del Valle- March 2005 to present.
- Medical Director Colombia Medical Mission – Hands Across The Americas. 2006 – 2007.
- Director of The Institute for Cancer Care, Mercy Medical Center, February 2006 – present.
- Chief of Surgical Oncology, Mercy Medical Center, February 2006 – present.
- Member of the Scientific Council of Colombia Médica-Universidad del Valle - 2005 to present.
- Member of the Scientific Review Committee, Mercy Medical Center – 2006 to 2011
- Medical Director Annual Colombia Medical Mission – 2006 to present
- Director of The Institute for Cancer Care, Mercy Medical Center, February 2006 to present

- Chief of Surgical Oncology, Mercy Medical Center, February 2006 to present
- The Commission on Cancer's Cancer Liaison Physician, January 2008 to present
- Member of Editorial Board of Colombia Médica - Universidad del Valle - 2009 to present
- Founder and President, Partners for Cancer Care and Prevention, Fundación Prevención y Tratamiento del Cáncer en Cali-Colombia – 2011 to present

HOSPITAL COMMITTEES
Ochsner Medical Institutions
Operating Room, 1992-1993
Oncology, 1989-1993
Pre-Operative Testing, 1992-1993

Health Care International (Scotland),Ltd.
Oncology, 1993-1994
Patient Education, 1993-1994
Drug and Therapeutics, 1993-1994
Clinical Systems Users, 1993-1994

St. Agnes HealthCare
Cancer Committee, 1994 - 2006
Patient Education, 1994 - 1997
Institutional Review Board, 1994 - 2006
Clinical Research Board of Directors, 1998 – 2006

Mercy Medical Center
Director of Institute for Cancer Care 2006 - present

Cancer Committee, 2006 - present
Cancer Liaison Physician, January 2008 - present

PRESENTATIONS

Sardi A, Gokli A, Singer J. Diverticular disease of the cecum and ascending colon: A review of 881 cases. Poster presentation, Southeastern Surgical Congress, New Orleans, LA, March 16-19, 1986

Sardi A, Parikh K, Singer J, Minken S. Mesenteric cysts. Poster presentation, Southeastern Surgical Congress, New Orleans, LA, March 16-19, 1986

Sardi A, Gokli A, Singer J. Diverticular disease of the cecum and ascending colon: A review of 881 cases. Presented at surgical grand rounds, Saint Agnes Hospital, Baltimore, MD, June 11, 1986

Sardi A, Rousseau M, Gersman M, Hinkle GH, Olsen J, Tuttle SE, Houchens D, Thurston MO, Martin EW Jr. Localization of tumor labeled with antibody 'cocktail' by hand-held gamma probe. Poster presentation, American Society of Colon and Rectal Surgeons, Washington DC, April 1987

Sickle-Santanello BJ, O'Dwyer PJ, Mojzisik CM, Tuttle SE, Hinkle GH, Rousseau M, Schlom J, Colcher D, Thurston MO, Nieroda C, **Sardi A**, Farrar WB, Minton JP, Martin EW Jr. Radioimmunoguided surgery using the monoclonal antibody B72.3 in colorectal tumors. Presented to the American Society of Colon and Rectal Surgeons Annual Meeting, Washington, DC, April 5-10, 1987

Siddiqi MA, Hinkle GH, Hill TL, Mojzisik CM, Olsen J, Rousseau M, Gersman M, Houchens D, **Sardi A**, Thurston MO, Martin EW Jr. An assessment of prolonged reactivity of seven monoclonal antibodies against in situ CX-1 tumor xenografts using a novel hand-held gamma detecting probe. Presented at the Third Annual Scientific Session of the Academy of Surgical Research, Washington, DC, September 10-12, 1987

Nieroda CA, Farrar WB, Mojzisik CM, **Sardi A**, Siddiqi MA, Ferrara PJ, Tuttle SE, James A, Martin E. A phase I study of the intraoperative detection of residual and metastatic breast cancer. Presented at the 10th Annual San Antonio Breast Cancer Symposium, San Antonio, TX, December 11-12, 1987

Sardi A, Siddiqi MA, Hinkle GH, Rousseau M, Gersman M, Hill TL, Olsen J, Tuttle SE, Young D, Houchens D, Thurston MO, Martin EW Jr. Localization of tumor labeled with antibody 'cocktail' by hand-held gamma probe. Presented at the 33rd Annual Meeting of the Ohio Chapter of American College of Surgeons, Resident Essay Contest, Akron, OH, May 5-7, 1988. First place winner Resident Essay contest and Extraordinary Oncology Award Winner.

Sardi A, Workman M, Mojzisik CM, Hinkle GH, Nieroda CA, Ferrara PJ, Agnone C, Farrar WB, Martin EW Jr. Intra-abdominal recurrence of colorectal cancer detected by radioimmunoguided surgery (RIGS). Presented at the 1988 Annual Meeting of the Society of Surgical Oncology, New Orleans, LA, May 22-25, 1988

Sardi A, Minton JP, Mojzisik CM, Nieroda CA, Ferrara PJ, Thurston MO, Martin EW Jr. The use of a hand-held gamma detector improves the safety of isolated limb perfusion. Poster presentation, 1988 Annual Meeting of the Society of Surgical Oncology, New Orleans, LA, May 22-25, 1988

Sardi A, Workman M, Mojzisik CM, Hinkle GH, Nieroda CA, Martin EW Jr. Intraabdominal recurrence of colorectal cancer detected by radioimmunoguided surgery (RIGS) system. Presented in the 1988 Annual Meeting of the Society of Surgical Oncology, New Orleans, LA, May 24, 1988

Nieroda CA, Mojzisik C, **Sardi A**, Ferrara PJ, Hinkle GH, Thurston MO, Martin EW Jr. The impact of radioimmunoguided surgery (RIGS) on surgical decision-making in colorectal cancer. Presented at the 1988 Annual Meeting of the American Society of Colon and Rectal Surgeons, Anaheim, CA, June 12-17, 1988

Ferrara PJ, Hinkle GH, Nieroda CA, **Sardi A**, Hill TL, Thurston M, Martin E. A dual-labeled monoclonal antibody allows radioimmunodetection (RID) and radioimmunoguided surgery (RIGS). Presented at the 1988 Annual Meeting of the American Society of Colon and Rectal Surgeons, Anaheim, CA, June 12-17, 1988

Sardi A, Agnone C, Nieroda CA, Mojzisik CM, Hinkle GH, Ferrara PJ, Farrar WB, Bolton J, Thurston MO, Martin E Jr. Radioimmunoguided surgery in recurrent colorectal cancer: The role of CEA, CAT scan, and physical examination. Presented in the Section of Colorectal Surgery at the 82nd Annual Scientific Assembly of the Southern Medical Association, New Orleans, LA, November 6-9, 1988

Sardi A, Radioimmunoguided surgery. Presented at the Association of Surgical Technologists of Louisiana Meeting, New Orleans, LA, February 1, 1989

Sardi A. Radioimmunoguided surgery. Presented at Ochsner Clinic Baton Rouge Satellite, Baton Rouge, LA, February 28, 1989

Sardi A. Surgical approach to recurrent colorectal cancer. Presented at North Central Cancer Treatment Group Meeting, Rochester, MN, April 5-7, 1989

Nieroda CA, Mojzisik C, Ferrara PJ, **Sardi A**, Hinkle GH, Thurston MO, Martin EW Jr. Radioimmunoguided surgery in primary colon cancer. Presented at the 3rd International Symposium on Immunobiology in Clinical Oncology, Nice France, April 9-11, 1989

Sardi A, Agnone C, Anderson G, Bolton JS, Sundgaard-Riise K, Nieroda CA, Minton JP. Low dose cyclophosphamide enhances helper-to-non-helper ratios. Presented at the 3rd International Symposium on Immunobiology in Clinical Oncology, Nice France, April 9-11, 1989

Sardi A, Martin EW Jr. The use of radioimmunoguided surgery in resecting retroperitoneal recurrent colorectal cancer. Presented in video form at the 1989 Meeting of the Society of Surgical Oncology, San Francisco, CA, May 21-24, 1989

Nieroda CAA, Agnone C, **Sardi A**, Houchens D, Hinkle GH, Bondo S, Martin EW Jr. Comparison of biokinetics of first and second generation monoclonal antibodies. Presented to the 80th Annual Meeting of the American Association for Cancer Research (AACR), May 24-27, 1989

Sardi A. Radioimmunoguided surgery. Presented at the Tulane University, New Orleans, LA, June 7, 1989

Sardi A. Recurrent colorectal cancer. Presented at Universidad del Valle, Cali, Colombia, July 14, 1989

Sardi A. Management of oral cavity cancer. Presented at the 1989 National Symposium of Surgery, San Salvador, El Salvador, September 21-24, 1989

Sardi A. Management of metastatic tumor to the neck with unknown primary. Presented at the 1989 National Symposium of Surgery, San Salvador, El Salvador, September 21-24, 1989

Sardi A. Management of carcinoma of the breast. Presented at the 1989 National Symposium of Surgery, San Salvador, El Salvador, September 21-24, 1989

Sardi A. Management of salivary gland tumors. Presented at the 1989 National Symposium of Surgery, San Salvador, El Salvador, September 21-24, 1989

Sardi A. The use of radioimmunoguided surgery in resecting retroperitoneal recurrent colorectal cancer. Presented in video form at the 1989 meeting of the American College of Surgeons, Atlanta, GA, October 15-20, 1989

Sardi A. Metastatic tumor to the neck with unknown primary. Presented at the XI Congreso de Actualización Médica, Cirugía y Especialidades, Guayaquil Ecuador, November 20-25, 1989

Sardi A. Oral cavity cancer. Presented at the XI Congreso de Actualización Médica, Cirugía y Especialidades, Guayaquil Ecuador, November 20-25, 1989

Sardi A. Surgical management of recurrent colorectal cancer. Presented at the XI Congreso de Actualización Médica, Cirugía y Especialidades, Guayaquil Ecuador, November 20-25, 1989

Sardi A. Advances in post-surgical adjuvant therapy for colon cancer: Results of recent NCCTG studies. Presented at the annual Joint Meeting of the Louisiana Chapter of the American College of Surgeons and the Surgical Association of Louisiana, New Orleans, LA, January 20-21, 1990

Sardi A. Management of in-situ breast cancer. Presented to sessions of the Update in Surgical Oncology - Use of the Cavitron (CUSA) and Intraoperative Ultrasound program, Louisiana

State University Medical Center, New Orleans, LA, April 26-27, 1990

Sardi A. New concepts in the surgical management of metastatic colorectal cancer - radioimmunoguided surgery - isolated hyperthermic liver perfusion. Made presentation as Director of course entitled "Current Management of Gastrointestinal Malignancies," Ochsner Foundation Hospital, New Orleans, LA, May 3-4, 1990

Sardi A. Surgical management of gastric lymphoma. Made presentation as Director of course entitled "Current Management of Gastrointestinal Malignancies," Ochsner Foundation Hospital, New Orleans, LA, May 3-4, 1990

Sardi A. Surgical management of recurrent colorectal cancer. Made presentation as invited Spring Visiting Professor at St. Agnes Hospital in Baltimore, MD, May 16, 1990

Sardi A. Walters P. DDS. A modified mandibular swing procedure for resection of carcinoma of the oropharynx. (Video). Presented to the Society of Head & Neck Surgeons, Washington DC, May 20-22, 1990

Martin EW Jr, Cohen AM, Lavery IC, Daly JM, **Sardi A,** Aitken D, Bland KI, Hinkle GH. Radioimmunoguided surgery: a preliminary report of a multicenter trial to evaluate the use of the radiolabeled B72.3 monoclonal antibody in colorectal cancer. Presented to the Society of Head & Neck Surgeons, Washington DC, May 20-22, 1990

Sardi A, Eckholdt G, McKinnon W, Bolton J. The significance of mammography changes following breast preservation for carcinoma of the breast. Poster presentation to the Society of Surgical Oncology, Washington DC, May 20-22, 1990

Sardi A, Merritt C, McKinnon W, Mitchell W, Bolton J, DeVun D, Troy D. Stereotactic guidance for breast biopsy localization and aspiration. Presented to the Society of Surgical Oncology, Washington DC, May 20-22, 1990

Cohen AM, Martin EW Jr, Lavery I, Daly J, **Sardi A**, Aitken D, Bland K, Mojzisik CM, Hinkle GH. Radioimmunoguided surgery using iodine 1251 B72.3 in patients with colorectal cancer. Presented to the 43rd Annual Cancer Symposium of the Society of Surgical Oncology, Washington, DC, May 21, 1990

Sardi A, Facundus E, Eckholdt G, McKinnon W, Bolton J. Management of cancer of the opposite breast following breast preservation. Presented to the 15th International Cancer Congress, Hamburg Germany, August 16-22, 1990

Sardi A, Walters P. DDS. A modified mandibular swing procedure for resection of carcinoma of the oropharynx. (Video). Presented to the American College of Surgeons, Clinical Congress, San Francisco, CA, October 7-12, 1990

Sardi A, Eckholdt G, McKinnon W, Bolton J. The significance of mammography changes following breast preservation for carcinoma of the breast. Presented to the 84th Annual Scientific

Assembly of the Southern Medical Association, Nashville, TN, October 14-17, 1990

Lavery I, Aitken D, **Sardi A**, Daly J, Bland K, Cohen A, Martin EW Jr. Phase I/II clinical study: the intraoperative detection of colorectal cancer by radiolabeled B72.3 monoclonal antibody. Presented at the 3rd Conference on Radioimmunodetection and Radioimmunotherapy of Cancer, Princeton, NJ, November 15-17, 1990

Sardi A. The use of radioimmunoguided surgery in resecting retroperitoneal recurrent colorectal cancer. Presented in video form at the International College of Surgeons, 1991 Annual Meeting, Williamsburg, VA, March 20-24, 1991

Sauter E, **Sardi A**. Prognostic Value of DNA Flow Cytometry in Parangliomas of the Head and Neck. Presented to the 84th Annual Scientific Assembly of the Southern Medical Association, Nashville, TN, October 14-17, 1990

Sardi A. Head and neck cancer. Presented at Tulane University Medical Center, New Orleans, LA, April 1, 1991

Sardi A. Surgical treatment of recurrent colorectal carcinoma. Presented to the Section of Family Medicine, Ochsner Clinic, New Orleans, LA, April 3, 1991

Sardi A. Significance of mammography and clinical findings following conservative surgery and radiation. Presented at the

Current Concepts in Oncology program at Ochsner Foundation Hospital, New Orleans, LA, April 25-26, 1991

Sardi A, Bolton J, Mitchell, W, Merritt C. Immunoperoxidase confirmation of ultrasonic-guided fine needle aspirates in patients with recurrent hyperparathyroidism. Presented at the Society of Head and Neck Surgeons, Annual Meeting, Maui, Hawaii, May 1-4, 1991

Sardi A, Skenderis B. Sisson procedure for resection of carcinoma of the thyroid. Presented at the Society of Head and Neck Surgeons, Annual Meeting, Maui, Hawaii, May 1-4, 1991

Sardi A. Surgical management of recurrent colorectal carcinoma. Presented at Surgical Grand Rounds at Tulane University Medical Center, New Orleans, LA, May 11, 1991

Sardi A. Surgical management of recurrent colorectal carcinoma. Presented to the Association of Surgical Technologists 23rd Annual National Conference, New Orleans, LA, June 26-29, 1991

Sardi A. Program Director for the Spring and Fall meetings of the New Orleans Surgical Society held at Ochsner Foundation Hospital, May 25, 1991, and Tulane University September 20-21, 1991

Sardi A. Head and Neck Surgery presented at the General Surgery Review Course of the Osler Institute in as mock oral exam preparation with didactic lecture in New Orleans, Louisiana, February 22, 1991; in Pittsburgh, Pennsylvania, September 21, 1991; in Seattle, Washington, June 7, 1991; and in Jacksonville, FL, December 14, 1991

Sardi A. Management of carcinoma in situ of the breast. Presented at the Fundación Santa Fe de Bogota, Cancer Institute Ardila Lulle, Bogota, Colombia, October 4, 1991

Sardi A. Surgical management of recurrent cancer of the colon and rectum. Presented at the Fundación Sante Fe de Bogota, Cancer Institute Ardila Lulle, Bogota, Colombia, October 4, 1991

Sardi A. Immunodirected surgery of metastatic colon carcinoma. Presented at La Academia Nacional de Medicina y Exposalud, Bogota, Colombia, October 5, 1991

Sardi A. Management of carcinoma in situ of the breast. Presented at the University Hospital, Cali, Colombia, October 7, 1991

Sardi A. Surgical management of recurrent cancer of the colon and rectum. Presented at the Universidad del Valle, Cali, Colombia, October 7, 1991

Sardi A. Current management of breast cancer. Presented at the Primary Care of the Hispanic American, Symposium #1, New Orleans, LA, October 24-26, 1991

Sardi A, Skenderis B. Sisson procedure for resection of carcinoma of the thyroid. Presented at the American College of Surgeons, 1991 Annual Meeting, Chicago, IL, October 20-25, 1991

Sardi A. Total pelvic exenteration with or without sacral resection in patients with recurrent rectal carcinoma. Presented at the 85th Scientific Assembly of the Southern Medical Association and the Medical Association of Georgia, Atlanta, GA, November 16-19, 1991

Sardi A. ^{111}In-CYT-103 used in research study. Presented at the Avance en la Detección y Seguimiento del Carcinoma Colorectal, Madrid Spain, December 12, 1991

Sardi A, Skenderis B. Sisson procedure for resection of carcinoma of the thyroid. Presented at the International College of Surgeons Annual Meeting, Chicago, IL, April 9-12, 1992

Sardi A, Finger I, Riggs P, Guerra L, Block M, Walters P. Radiated bone and implants. Presented to the Third International Conference on Head and Neck Cancer, San Francisco, CA, July 1992

Sardi A. Laparoscopic hernia repair. Presented at the training course. Panama City, Panama, July 23 - 25, 1992

Sardi A. Laparoscopic hernia repair. Presented at the training course. Fundacion Santa Fe, Bogota, Colombia, July 27, 1992

Sardi A. Laparoscopic hernia repair. Presented at the training course. Universidad del Valle, Cali, Colombia, July 28, 1992 and August 6, 1992

Sardi A. The Use of Radioimmunoguided surgery in resection retroperitoneal recurrent colorectal cancer. Presented at 1992 Clinical Congress of the American College of Surgeons, October 11-16, 1992

Sardi A, Weiss C. Clinical prognostic factors in patients with metastatic carcinoma with unknown primary. Presented at the 86th Annual Scientific Assembly, Southern Medical Association, San Antonio, TX, November 12-15, 1992

Sardi A, Facundus E, Bergeron R, Bolton J. Breast Hamartomas: Selective management following mammographic diagnosis. Poster presentation at the 15th Annual San Antonio Breast Cancer Symposium, San Antonio, Texas, December 9-10, 1992

Sardi A, Skenderis B, Hoffmann B, Bolton J, Willis G. Ploidy status predicts survival in patients with gastric lymphoma. Presented at the Southeastern Surgical Congress, Tarpon Springs, FL, February 7-11, 1993

Sardi, A. Advances in laparoscopic surgery: Splenectomy, adrenalectomy, hernia. Presented at the 2nd Congress of Private Hospitals of Guatemala, Guatemala City, Guatemala, March 11-13, 1993

Sardi A, Witherspoon L, Bolton J, Farr G, Hicks T, Gathright J. Monoclonal antibody ^{111}In-CYT-103 improves detection and management of recurrent colorectal cancer. Presented at The Society of Surgical Oncology meeting, Los Angeles, CA, March 18-21, 1993

Sardi, A. Laparoscopic aplenectomy for a patient with idiopathic thrombocytopenic purpura. Presented at the 46th annual Cancer Symposium of the Society of Surgical Oncology, Los Angeles, CA, March 18-21, 1993

Sardi A. Advanced laparoscopic applications. Presented at the Association of Surgical Technologists meeting, New Orleans, LA, March 27, 1993

Sardi, A. Cirugía laparoscópica su desarrollo y últimos avances. XV Aniversario Fundación, Hospital de Diagnóstico, San Salvador, El Salvador, March 30-April 2, 1993

Sardi, A. Recurrent colorectal carcinoma. Timing and extent of operation: Do they make a difference? Presented at Advances in the Diagnosis and Management of Colorectal and Ovarian Carcinoma, Puerto Vallarta Mexico, April 22-26, 1993

Sardi, A. Monoclonal antibodies in the treatment of recurrent colorectal carcinoma. Presented at Oncology Conference of Morton Plant Hospital, Clearwater, FL, May 13, 1993

Sardi, A. Manejo Actual del Cáncer Gástrico. Presented at XVII Congreso Nacional de Cirugía, Cuenca Ecuador, May 25-26, 1993

Sardi, A. Laparoscopic splenectomy for a patient with idiopathic thrombocytopenic purpura. Presented at Laparoscopic Procedures Course held at Universidad del Valle, Cali, Colombia; May 28, 1993

Sardi, A. Laparoscopic splenectomy for a patient with idiopathic thrombocytopenic purpura. Presented at XVII Congreso Nacional de Cirugía, Cuenca Ecuador, May 25-26, 1993

Sardi A. Advanced laparoscopic techniques: Colon resection small bowel, resection highly selective vagotomy, adrenalectomy, and splenectomy. Presented at Hospital Universitario del Valle, Cali, Colombia; May 27-28, 1993

Sardi, A. Estado actual de cirugía laparoscopica. Presented at XVII Congreso Nacional de Cirugía, Cuenca Ecuador, May 25-26, 1993

Sardi, A. Colecistectomia por laparoscopia. Presented at XVII Congreso Nacional de Cirugía, Cuenca, Ecuador, May 25-26, 1993

Sardi, A. Problemas durante cirugía laparoscópica. Presented at XVII Congreso Nacional de Cirugía, Cuenca Ecuador, May 25-26, 1993

Sardi A. Monoclonal antibodies in the management of recurrent colorectal cancer. Presented at Palm Beach Gardens Imaging Center, Palm Beach Gardens, FL, July 30, 1993

Sardi A. The surgical management of recurrent colorectal cancer: The role of monoclonal antibodies. Presented at Massapequa General Hospital, Seaport, NY, August 18, 1993

Sardi A. The surgical management of recurrent colorectal cancer: The role of monoclonal antibodies. Presented at Long Island College Hospital, Long Island, New York, August 18, 1993

Sardi A. McKinnon W. Laparoscopic left adrenalectomy for primary aldosteronism. Presented at the 17th Annual Conference at American College of Surgeons, San Francisco, CA, October 10-15, 1993

Sardi, A. Radical nephrectomy and partial resection of inferior vena cava with extraction of tumor thrombus in renal cell carcinoma. Presented at American College of Surgeons, San Francisco, CA, October 10-15, 1993

Sardi, A. Laparoscopic splenectomy for a patient with idiopathic thrombocytopenic purpura. Presented at the 4th World Congress International Gastro-Surgical Club in Madrid Spain, October 29, 1993

Sardi, A. McKinnon W. Laparoscopic left adrenalectomy for primary aldosteronism. Presented at the 4th World Congress International Gastro-Surgical Club in Madrid Spain, October 29, 1993

Sardi, A. Present status of surgical management of recurrent colorectal cancer. Presented at "Theagenion" Cancer Institute in Thessaloniki Greece, November 16, 1993

Sardi, A. Current status of laparoscopic surgery. Presented at the Aristotelion University of Thessaloniki Medical School, Thessaloniki Greece, November 17, 1993

Sardi, A. Current status of laparoscopic surgery. Presented at Athens University Medical School, Athens Greece, November 18, 1983

Sardi, A. Current status of laparoscopic surgery. Presented at the 1st International Aesculapean Seminar on Female Urology, University of Patras Greece, November 20, 1993

Sardi, A. Surgical aspects of breast cancer. Presented in Cairo Egypt, December 13, 1993

Sardi, A. The surgical management of recurrent colorectal cancer. Presented in Cairo Egypt, December 13, 1993

Sardi, A. Laparoscopic assisted small bowel resection. Presented at the International meeting of surgery, Madrid Spain, May 23 1994

Sardi, A. Surgical management of recurrent colorectal cancer. Presented at XVII International meeting of surgery, Madrid Spain, May 24, 1994

Sardi, A. Laparoscopic right and left adrenalectomy. Presented at International meeting of surgery, Madrid Spain, May 24, 1994

Sardi, A. Management of special problems during laparoscopic cholecystectomy. Presented at XVII International meeting of surgery, Madrid Spain, May 26, 1994

Sardi, A. Gastric cancer; What's new in 1994. Presented at XVII International meeting of surgery, Madrid Spain, May 27, 1994

Sardi, A. Management of carcinoma in situ of the Breast. Presented at XVII International meeting of surgery, Madrid Spain, May 28, 1994

Sardi, A. Surgical techniques for tumors. Presented at Symposium on Recent Advances in Cancer Management, Cairo Egypt, June 27, 1994

Sardi, A. Management of oral cavity cancer. Medical Grand Rounds, Health Care International, Glasgow Scotland, July 6, 1994

Sardi, A. Management of oral cavity cancer. Surgical Grand Rounds. Saint Agnes Hospital. Baltimore, MD, September 14, 1994

Sardi, A. Bilateral laparoscopic lumbar sympathectomy. Presented at the 80th Congress of the American College of Surgeons, Chicago, IL, October 11, 1994

Sardi, A. Cervical lymph node metastasis. Surgical Grand Rounds, North Arundel Hospital, Baltimore, MD, November 17, 1994

Sardi, A. Cervical lymph node metastasis. Medical Grand Rounds, St. Agnes Hospital, Baltimore, MD, January 26, 1995

Sardi, A. Manejo del cáncer gastrico. Fundacion Valle del Lili, Primer Simposio de Cancer, Cali, Colombia, February 23, 1995

Sardi, A. Manejo del cáncer esofágico. Fundacion Valle del Lili, Primer Simposio de Cancer, Cali, Colombia, February 24, 1995

Sardi, A. Técnicas quirúrgicas en el cáncer primario y metastático del hígado. Fundacion Valle del Lili, Primer Simposio de Cancer, Cali, Colombia, February 23, 1995

Sardi, A. Surgical management of recurrent colorectal cancer: The role of monoclonal antibodies. Maryland Association of Nuclear Medicine Technology, St. Joseph Hospital, Baltimore, MD, April 26, 1995

Sardi A. Surgery in Cancer: U.S.-Colombian Medical Association XV Congress New Orleans, LA, July 27- 29, 1995

Sardi A. Surgical influences in quality of life. St Agnes Hospital Medical Grand Rounds. Baltimore, MD, September 14, 1995

Sardi A. Liver metastasis. St Agnes Hospital Department of Medicine. Baltimore, MD, November 7, 1995

Pergolizzi J Jr, **Sardi A**, Pelzar M. Merkel Cell carcinoma: An aggressive malignancy. Presented at the 64 Annual Scientific Meeting, Southeastern Surgical Congress, Tampa FL, February 3-7 1996

Sardi A. Surgical management of recurrent colorectal cancer. Presented at Surgical Grand Rounds. Harbor Hospital Baltimore, MD, February 15, 1996

Sardi A Management of Sarcomas. Presented at Surgical Grand Rounds. Mercy Hospital Baltimore, MD, February 29, 1996

Sardi A Surgical management of recurrent colorectal cancer: Role of monoclonal antibodies. Presented at the Maryland Association of Nuclear Medicine Technology. Bethesda, MD, September 28th 1996

Cervone A, **Sardi A.**, Conaway G. Intraoperative ultrasound is essential in the management of metastatic liver lesions. Presented at the 82nd Annual Clinical Congress of the American College of Surgeons, San Francisco, CA, October 6-11, 1996

Ehrmantraut W , **Sardi A.** Laparoscopic small bowel resection. Presented at the 82nd Annual Clinical Congress of the American College of Surgeons, San Francisco, CA, October 6-11, 1996

Pergolizzi J Jr, **Sardi A,** Bolton J. A prospective randomized study of percutaneous placed versus external jugular venous cut down for long-term venous access. Presented at the 82nd

Annual Clinical Congress of the American College of Surgeons, San Francisco, CA, October 6-11, 1996

Stancofski E, **Sardi A**, Conaway G. Successful outcome in Swan-Ganz catheter induced rupture of pulmonary artery. Presented at the SouthEastern Surgical Congress, 65th Annual Scientific Meeting, Nashville, TN, February 3 - 5, 1997

Akbarov A, **Sardi A**, Conaway G, Spiegler E, Pelczar M, Roffe M. Radioimmunoguided surgery (RIGS) for patients with intraabdominal metastatic carcinoma of the colon and rectum. Presented at the SouthEastern Surgical Congress, 65th Annual Scientific Meeting, Nashville, TN, February 3 - 5, 1997

Sardi A, Layne E. Hemicorporectomy in a patient with squamous cell carcinoma arising from a sacral decubitus ulcer (Marjolin's ulcer). Video presented at the 83rd Annual Clinical Congress of the American College of Surgeons, Chicago, Illinois 1997

Sardi A, Sisson procedure for resection of carcinoma of the thyroid. Presented at Greater Baltimore Medical Center. Third Annual Darrell A. Jacques Symposium, Baltimore, MD.

Ehrmantraut W Jr, **Sardi A**, Singer J, Spiegler E. Review of Sestamibi technetium scan for detection of parathyroid adenoma. Presented at the 66th Annual Scientific Meeting of the Southeastern Surgical Congress, Atlanta, GA, February 2-5, 1998

Moran J, **Sardi A**, Keramati B. Retrosternal goiter: An unusual radiologic presentation. Presented at the 66th Annual Scientific Meeting of the Southeastern Surgical Congress, Atlanta, GA, February 2-5, 1998

Moran J, **Sardi A**, Singer J. Retrosternal goiter. Presented at the 66th Annual Scientific Meeting of the Southeastern Surgical Congress, Atlanta, GA, February 2-5, 1998

Ojeda H, **Sardi A**. Laparoscopic treatment of a true cyst of the spleen producing high levels of CEA and CA 19-9. Presented at the 66th Annual Scientific Meeting of the Southeastern Surgical Congress, Atlanta, GA, February 2-5, 1998

Sardi A, Management of primary and metastatic tumors to the liver. Presented at Surgical Grand Rounds, Washington Hospital Center, Washington DC, February 24, 1998

Sardi A. Minimally invasive procedures in the management of cancer. Internal Medicine Grand Rounds. St. Agnes HealthCare, Baltimore, MD, September 10, 1998

Singh K, **Sardi A**, Cotton B. Hemicorporectomy for patients with squamous cell carcinoma in chronic pressure ulcers - a review. Presented at 84th Annual Clinical Congress of the American College of Surgeons, Orlando, FL, October 25-30, 1998

Stone M, **Sardi A**, Conaway, G. Safe performance of major hepatic resection in a community hospital. Presented at 84th

Annual Clinical Congress of the American College of Surgeons, Orlando, FL, October 25-30, 1998

Heeringa B, **Sardi A**. Bleeding hepatic adenoma; expectant treatment to limit the extent of liver resection. Presented at 84th Annual Clinical Congress of the American College of Surgeons, Orlando, FL, October 25-30, 1998

Ojeda H, **Sardi A**. Male breast cancer: A 12-year review study of 16 cases with an unusual rate of secondary malignancies. Presented at 84th Annual Clinical Congress of the American College of Surgeons, Orlando, FL, October 25-30, 1998

Sardi A, Ojeda H. Laparoscopic treatment of true cyst of the spleen producing high levels of CEA and CA19-9. Video presented in the general surgical section at the 84th annual clinical congress of the American College of Surgeons. Orlando, FL, October 25-30, 1998

Sardi A. Sentinel node biopsy for breast cancer and melanoma. Presented at the Mid-Eastern Chapter of the Society of Nuclear Medicine. National Institute of Health, Bethesda, MD, November 4, 1998

Sardi A. Management of sarcoma. Presented at Surgical grand rounds. St. Agnes HealthCare. Baltimore, MD, November 18, 1998

Sardi A. Minimally invasive procedures in the management of cancer. Presented at OB-Gyn grand rounds. St. Agnes HealthCare. Baltimore, MD, November 18, 1998

Sardi A. Sentinel lymph node in breast cancer and melanoma. Presented at Centro Medico Imbanaco. Cali, Colombia, December 18, 1998

Ojeda H, **Sardi A.** Cryosurgery: adjuvant treatment at the time of resection of a pelvic recurrence in rectal cancer. Presented at the 67th annual meeting of the Southeastern Surgical Congress. Tampa, FL, February 15, 1999

Sardi A. Sentinel breast mapping in melanoma and breast cancer. Presented at Frederick Memorial Hospital. Frederick, MD, February 19, 1999

Sardi A. Sentinel breast mapping in melanoma and breast cancer. Presented at Surgical Grand Rounds St. Joseph Medical Center. Baltimore, MD, March 5, 1999

Sardi A. Sentinel node mapping in breast cancer and utilization of breast imaging with mammoscintigraphy. Presented in San Diego, CA DuPont Pharmaceuticals Clinical Specialist Groups, March 17, 1999

Sardi A. Management of breast cancer. Presented in San Diego CA DuPont Pharmaceuticals Clinical Specialist Groups, March 17, 1999

Sardi A. Sentinel lymph node mapping in breast cancer and melanoma. Presented for Central Pennsylvania Nuclear Medicine Technologist Association. Harrisburg, PA, March 25, 1999

Sardi A. Sentinel lymph node mapping in breast cancer and melanoma. Presented at Harbor Hospital. Baltimore, MD, April 15, 1999

Ojeda H, **Sardi A,** Cotton B, Pelczar M. Adenosquamous cell carcinoma of the breast with recurrent metastases of squamous cell component: An unusual aggressive presentation. Presented at the 85th Congress of American College of Surgeons Clinical Congress, San Francisco, CA, October 11-14, 1999

Averbach A, **Sardi A,** Ottaviano Y, Conaway G. Cytoreductive surgery with perioperative intraperitoneal chemotherapy for peritoneal carcinomatosis in a community teaching hospital. Presented at the 85th Congress of the American College of Surgeons Clinical Congress, San Francisco, CA, October 11-14, 1999

McMasters KM, Wong SL, Tuttle TM, Carlson DJ, Brown CM, Noyes RD, Glaser, RL, Vennekotter DJ, Turk PS, Tate PS, **Sardi A**, Edwards MJ. Sentinel lymph node (SLN) biopsy for breast cancer. Obtaining a preoperative lymphoscintigram does not improve SLN identification or false-negative rates. Presented at the Southern Surgical Association, Hot Springs, VA, December 5-8, 1999

Sardi A. The benefit of using two techniques for sentinel lymph node mapping in breast cancer. Presented at 68th annual meeting of the Southeastern Surgical Congress, Lake Buena Vista, FL, February 6-8, 2000

Sardi A, Kunjummen B, Rehman S, Spiegler E, Colandrea J, Frishberg D, Singh H, Regan P, Totoonchie A, Merchant D. The impact of using two techniques in SLN mapping for breast cancer. Presented at the 10th Congress of the European Society of Surgical Oncology. Groningen Netherlands, April 5-8, 2000

Sardi A. Aggressive cytoreductive surgery and hyperthermic intraoperative intraperitoneal chemotherapy in advanced intraperitoneal malignancies - A pilot study. Presented at the Millenium Master class The Royal College of Surgeons of England. London England, June 1-2, 2000

Sardi A. Implementation of a protocol for aggressive cytoreductive surgery and hyperthermic intraoperative intraperitoneal chemotherapy in peritoneal carcinomatosis and sarcomatosis. Presented at the Milledium Master Class The Royal College of Surgeons of England. London England, June 1-2, 2000

Sardi A. Advances in the surgical therapy of breast cancer with emphasis on sentinel node biopsy. Presented at the XXth US-Colombian Medical Association Congress, Washington DC, July 8, 2000

Averbach A, Kunjummen B, Buscema J, Krishnaiah G, Conaway G, **Sardi A**. Cytoreductive surgery with perioperative intraperitoneal chemotherapy for peritoneal carcinomatosis of appendiceal, colonic, ovarian and mesothelial origin: Preliminary results of the phase I/II study. Poster Presentation at 69th annual meeting of the Southeastern Surgical Congress, New Orleans, LA, February 3-6, 2001

Kunjummen B, **Sardi A**. Safe early postoperative oral feeding after gastrointestinal surgery presented at 69th annual meeting of the Southeastern Surgical Congress, New Orleans, LA, February 3-6, 2001

Kunjummen B, **Sardi A**. Previous lumpectomy does not influence the sensitivity of sentinel lymph node mapping in breast cancer. Presented at 69th annual meeting of the Southeastern Surgical Congress, New Orleans, LA, February 3-6, 2001

Krishnaiah G, **Sardi A**, Kunjummen B, Regan P, Singer J, Totoonchie A, Spiegler E. Technetium-99M sestamibi scintimammography complements mammography in the detection of breast cancer. Presented at the 6th Annual Multidisciplinary Symposium on Breast Disease, Amelia Island, Florida, February 15-18, 2001

Ganti A, **Sardi A**, Gordon J. Laparoscopic treatment of large true cysts of liver and spleen is ineffective. Presented at the 70th Annual meeting of the Southeastern Surgical Congress. Nashville, TN, February 3-5, 2002

Averbach A, **Sardi A**, Sher-Ahmad A, Krishnaiah G, Buscema J, Bieligk S. Cytoreductive surgery with perioperative intraperitoneal chemotherapy for peritoneal carcinomatosis: A pilot study. Presented at The 55th Annual Congress of the Society of Surgical Oncology. Denver, CO, March 14-17, 2002

Gann M, **Sardi A**. Improved results using ultrasound guidance for central venous access. Presented at the 71st Annual meeting of the Southeastern Surgical Congress, Savannah, GA, February 7-11, 2003

Sardi A, Bieligk S. Early postoperative oral Intake in a surgical oncology practice. Presented at the 56th Annual Congress of the Surgical Oncology. Los Angeles, CA. March 2003

Sardi A. Intraductal approach to breast cancer in high-risk patients. Presented at OB/GYN Grand Rounds. St Agnes HealthCare, Baltimore, MD. September 17, 2003

Sardi A. Minimally invasive approaches in the management of breast cancer. Presented at Medical and Surgical Grand Rounds at Harbor Hospital. Baltimore MD. September 18,2003

Sardi A. Intraductal approach to breast cancer in high-risk patients. Presented at Medical Grand Rounds St Agnes HealthCare, Baltimore, MD. September 25, 2003

Sardi A. Aggressive Management of Peritoneal carcinomatosis. Present role of hyperthermic intraoperative intraperitoneal chemotherapy. Presented at The Surgical Grand Rounds North Arundel Hospital. Baltimore, MD. October 16, 2003

Green A, Fleming J, Ashfaq R, Rege R, **Sardi A**, Bieligk S. The utility of laparoscopic peritoneal cytology in patients with malignant disease confined to the abdomen. Presented at the annual congress of the American College of Surgeons, San Francisco, CA 2003

Sardi A. Sentinel lymph node biopsy in breast cancer. Presented at Centro Imbanaco, Cali, Colombia, December 29, 2003

Gann M, Merriman B, **Sardi A.** Safe performance of thyroid and parathyroid surgery in a community teaching hospital. Presented at the annual congress of the SouthEastern Surgical Society, Atlanta, GA. February 1-3, 2004

Peterson R, **Sardi A.** Hemicorporectomy: Seven years of follow up. Presented at the annual congress of the Southeastern Surgical Society, Atlanta, GA. February 1-3, 2004

Hamoudi D. **Sardi A**. Benayache I., Cianos R. Merriman, B. Improved long term survival following Cytoreductive Surgery and Intra-peritoneal Hyperthermic Chemotherapy for Peritoneal Carcinomatosis. Presented at the Congress of the American College Surgeons Clinical Congress. October 2004

Karpinski S, **Sardi A.** Thorascopic Resection of Mediastinal Intrathymic ParathyroidAdenoma: A case Report. Accepted for presentation to the Southeastern Surgical Congress, New Orleans 11-15, 2005

Stephenson S, **Sardi A.** Chest computer tomography for lung screening. Accepted for presentation to the Southeastern Surgical Congress, New Orleans, February 11-15 2005

Peterson R, **Sardi A.** Analytic Uncertainty and Clinical Impact of Human Growth Factor Reeceptor-2 (HER-2/neu) Testing in a

Community Hospital. Accepted for presentation to the Southeastern Surgical Congress, New Orleans, February 11-15 2005

Hamdalah I, **Sardi A.** Absence of the Retrohepatic Inferior Vena Cava-What the surgeon should know. Accepted for presentation to the Southeastern Surgical Congress, New Orleans, February 11-15 2005

Hamdalah I, **Sardi A.** Diagnostic Value of Preoperative FNA in Follicular and Hurthle Cell Neoplasms. Presented at the 58th Annual Cancer Symposium, Society of Surgical Oncology, Atlanta, February 2005

Sardi A. Management of Peritoneal Carcinomatosis. Presented at Fundacion Valle del Lili, Cali, Colombia. June 7, 2005

Sardi A. Intraperitoneal Hyperthermic Chemotherapy (IPHC) for the Treatment Abdominal Carcinomatosis: Indications and results. Presented at the Maryland Medical Convention, October 19, 2005

Sardi A. Intraperitoneal Hyperthermic Chemotherapy (IPHC) for the Treatment Abdominal Carcinomatosis: Indications and results. Presented at Mercy Medical Center, Baltimore, MD January 25, 2006

Bashir A, Bieligk S, Cadogan M, **Sardi A**. Scalp Angiosarcoma with Metastasis to the Lung Presenting as a Bleb. Presented to the Southeastern Surgical Congress Annual Scientific Meeting, February 2006

Mallalieu J, Marques M, **Sardi A.** Hyperbaric Oxygen Therapy in the Treatment of Radiation Enteritis: A Solution for a Debilitating Condition. Presented to the Southeastern Surgical Congress Annual Scientific Meeting, February 2006

Semino-Mora C, **Sardi A,** Liu H, McAvoy T, Dubois A. Pseudomyxoma Peritonei: An infectious disease? Presented at the 59th Annual Cancer Symposium, SSO, San Diego, CA, March 23-26, 2006

Franco G, Kostuik P, Nieroda CA, Cianos R, Merriman B, **Sardi A.** Impact of Cytoreductive Surgery and Hyperthermic Intraperitoneal Chemotherapy in Patients with Disseminated Intraabdominal Carcinomatosis. Presented at the 59th Annual Cancer Symposium, SSO, San Diego, CA, March 23-26, 2006

Sardi A. Surgical and Chemotherapeutic Management of Peritoneal Neoplasia. Presented at Advances in Gynecologic Oncology Symposium, Mercy Medical Center, Baltimore, MD, April 29, 2006

Sardi A. The management of liver metastasis. Presented at Surgical Grand Rounds, Mercy Medical Center, Baltimore, MD, May 11, 2006

Thillainathan V, Nieroda CA, Kostuik P, Merriman B, **Sardi A**. Comparison of Open and Closed Techniques of Delivery of Hyperthermic Chemotherapy following Cytoreductive Surgery in patients with Peritoneal Carcinomatosis. Presented at the American Society of Clinical Oncology Annual Meeting, Atlanta, GA, June 3, 2006

Baraki Y, **Sardi A.** Long Term Survival Following Cytoreductive Surgery and Intraperitoneal Hyperthermic Chemotherapy for Dissemenated Appendiceal Tumors. Presented at the American Society of Clinical Oncology Annual Meeting, Atlanta, GA, June 3, 2006

Sardi A. Current Changes in the Management of Peritoneal Carcinomatosis. Presented at the Symposium on Diagnosis and Treatment of Peritoneal Malignancy. Mercy Medical Center, Baltimore, MD, September 16, 2006

Munalula J, Thillainathan V, Nieroda CA, Kostuik P, Gushchin V, Holter D, Kalesan B, **Sardi A**. Comparison of Open and Closed Technique for Delivery of Hyperthermic Intraperitoneal Chemotherapy following Cytoreductive Surgery for Peritoneal Carcinomatosis. Presented at the Am College of Surgeons, Chicago, IL, October 8-12, 2006

Sardi A. Current Challenges in the Management of Peritoneal Carcinomatosis. Presented at National Nurses Oncology Education Day. Mercy Medical Center, Baltimore, MD, November 2, 2006

Sardi A. Tratamiento multidisciplinario de las metastasis hepáticas. Presented at the 16th Congreso Nacional de Cancerologia, Bogotá, Colombia, November 9-12, 2006

Sardi A. Melanoma. Tratamiento quirúrgico. Presented at the 16th Congreso Nacional de Cancerologia. Bogotá, Colombia, November 9-12, 2006

Sardi A. Tratamiento de la carcinomatosis peritoneal. Presented at the 16th Congreso Nacional de Cancerologia. Bogotá, Colombia, November 9-12, 2006

Kostuik P, Munalula J, Thillaniathan V, Nieroda CA, Gushchin V, Holter D, Kalesan B, **Sardi A.** Comparison of Open and Closed Technique for Delivery of Hyperthermic Intraperitoneal Chemotherapy following Cytoreductive Surgery for Peritoneal Carcinomatosis. Presented at the 5th International Workshop on Peritoneal Surface Malignancy, Milan, Italy, December 4-6, 2006

Sardi A. The Changing Paradigm in Surgical Oncology. Presented at Medical Grand Rounds. Mercy Medical Center, Baltimore, MD, January 31, 2007

Munalula J, Nieroda CA, Kostuik P, Holter D, Kalesan B, **Sardi A.** Aggressive Cytoreduction Surgery for Peritoneal Carcinomatosis with Low Incidences of Stoma Creation. Presented to the Southeastern Surgical Congress Annual Scientific Meeting, Savannah, GA, February 10-13, 2007

Hamdallah I, Ballo M, **Sardi A.** Lower Incidence of Coexistent Carcinoma in Patients with Atypical Ductal Hyperplasia on Stereotactic Breast Biopsy. Presented to the Southeastern

Surgical Congress Annual Scientific Meeting, Savannah, GA, February 10-13, 2007

Karras RA, **Sardi A.** Intra-Abdominal and Retroperitoneal Catecholamine Producing Paragangliomas. Presented to the Southeastern Surgical Congress Annual Scientific Meeting, Savannah, GA, February 10-13, 2007.

Karras RA, **Sardi A.** Concomitant Multi-Organ Cysts, Renal Cell Carcinoma and Pheochromocytoma in Von Hipple-Lindau Disease: A Case Report. Presented to the Southeasern Surgical Congress Annual Scientific Meeting, Savannah, GA, February 10-13, 2007

Munalula J, Nieroda CA, Kostuik P, Holter D, Kalesan B, Gushchin V, **Sardi A**. Cytoreductive surgery followed with in-traperitoneal hyperthermic chemotherapy in elder patients with appendiceal carcinomatosis. Presented to Society of Surgical Oncology 60th Annual Cancer Symposium, Washington, D.C., March 15-18, 2007

Sardi A. Multi-disciplinary Approach in the Treatment of Recurrent and Stage IV Colorectal Cancer: A Surgical Perspective. Presented at A Symposium on Diagnosis and Treatment of Gastrointestinal Malignancies. Mercy Medical Center, Baltimore, MD September 29, 2007

Gushchin V, Ross A, Miller D, Nieroda CA, Kalesan B, Studeman K, Kostuik P, **Sardi A**. Complete Cytoreduction Offers

Long-term Survival in Patients with Peritoneal Carcinomatosis from Appendiceal Tumors of Unfavorable Histology. Presented to the American College of Surgeons, San Francisco, CA, October 15, 2008.

Sardi A. Current Approach to Peritoneal Carcinomatosis of Gastrointestinal Origin. Presented at Symposium in the diagnosis and treatment of peritoneal malignancy. Mercy Medical Center, Baltimore MD, November 1, 2008.

Sardi A, Nieroda CA, Gushchin V. Approach to the porta hepaticus during cytoreductive surgery: Important technical considerations. Presented at the 6th International Workshop on Peritoneal Surface Malignancy, Lyone, France, November 17-19, 2008.

Nieroda CA, Jonas S, Kostuik P, **Sardi A.** The Role of Cytoreductive Surgery and Hyperthermic Intraperitoneal Chemotherapy in Recurrent Ovarian Cancer: A Case Study. Presented at the 2009 Southeastern Surgical Congress Annual Scientific Meeting, Atlanta, GA, February 7-9, 2009.

Sardi A. Cáncer al Colon. Presented at Taller Informativo De Cancer "Preguntele A Los Expertos." Johns Hopkins Bayview Medical Center, March 19, 2009.

Sardi A. Peritoneal carcinomatosis: Not the end of the road? Presented at the 1st Annual GI Symposium, Mercy Medical Center, Baltimore, MD. October 2, 2009

Sardi A, Omohwo C, Nieroda CA, Holter D, Athas N, Gushchin V. Bowel Complications in Patients with Peritoneal Carcinomatosis of Appendiceal Origen Treated with Cytoreductive Surgery and Hyperthermic Intraperitoneal Chemotherapy." Presented to Society of Surgical Oncology 63rd Annual Cancer Symposium, St. Louis, MO. March 3-7, 2010

Thieme H, Gushchin V, **Sardi A,** Athas N. Peritoneal Carcinomatosis in the Geriatric Patient: Outcomes with Cytoreductive Surgery and HIPEC. Presented to Society of Surgical Oncology 63rd Annual Cancer Symposium, St. Louis, MO, March 3-7, 2010

Sardi A. Treatment for Peritoneal Carcinomatosis. Presented to the PMP Research Foundation Inaugural Practitioner-Patient Symposium. Upland, PA June 19, 2010

Sardi A., Francis J, Marshall M, MacDonald R, Holter D, Gushchin V. Prophylactic IVC filters in patients undergoing Cytoreductive and Hyperthermic Intraperitoneal Chemotherapy (HIPEC). Presented at the 7th International Workshop on Peritoneal Surface Malignancies, Uppsala, Sweden, September 2010

Sardi A, Omohwo C, Nieroda CA, Holter D, Athas N, Gushchin V. Bowel Complications In Patients with Peritoneal Carcinomatosis of Appendiceal Origen Treated with Cytoreductive Surgery and Hyperthermic Intraperitoneal Chemotherapy. Presented at the 7th International Workshop on Peritoneal Surface Malignancies, Uppsala, Sweden, September 2010

Mitzel A, McBeth M, Appling S, MacDonald R, **Sardi A**. Intraoperative Upper Extremity Repositioning to Prevent Peripheral Neuropathy in Patients Undergoing Cytoreductive Surgery/Hyperthermic Intraperitoneal Chemotherapy (HIPEC): A Nursing Perspective. Presented at the 7th International Workshop on Peritoneal Surface Malignancies, Uppsala, Sweden, September 2010.

El Halabi H, Gushchin V, Macdonald R, Francis J, **Sardi A.** Patients with high-grade appendix cancer and extensive disease do benefit from Cytoreduction and heated intraperitoneal chemotherapy if complete cytoreduction can be achieved. Presented to Society of Surgical Oncology at 64th Annual Cancer Symposium, San Antonio, TX, March 2-5, 2011.

El Halabi H, Gushchin V, Macdonald R, Francis J, Athas N, **Sardi A.** Lymph node metastasis predicts survival in patients with high grade appendix cancer. Presented to Society of Surgical Oncology at 64th Annual Cancer Symposium, San Antonio, TX, March 2-5, 2011.

Sardi A. Peritoneal carcinomatosis: Not the end of the road. Presented at the Tumor Board at the University of Valle in Cali-Colombia, April 8, 2011.

El Halabi H, Ledakis P, Gushchin V, Francis J, Athas N, Macdonald R, Studeman K, **Sardi A.** The role of cytoreductive surgery in patients with carcinomatosis from high-grade appendix cancer in the era of modern systemic chemotherapy. Presented to ASCO Annual Meeting in Chicago, IL June 3-5, 2011

Sardi A. GI Neuroendocrine Tumors: A Team Approach. Presented to 3rd Annual Consensus and Controversies in Gastroenterology & Hepatology. Mercy Medical Center, Baltimore, MD September 23-24, 2011

Sardi A. Neuroendocrine Tumors: A Team Approach. Presented at Cancer Care: Back to Basics, A Comprehensive Look at A Multidisciplinary Approach in Treatment of Oncological Diseases. The Institute for Cancer Care at Mercy Medical Center, Baltimore, MD February 3, 2012

Wosu C, El-Halabi, Wong M, Gallagher B, Francis J, Studeman K, Ledakis P, Nieroda C, Gushchin V, **Sardi A.** Progression of Peritoneal Adenomucinosis to the Scrotum: A Rare Occurrence Treated with Cytoreductive Surgery and Hyperthermic Intraperitoneal Chemotherapy. Presented at the Seventh International Symposium on Regional Cancer Therapies, Captiva, Florida, February 18-20, 2012

El Halabi H, Gushchin V, Francis J, MacDonald R, Studeman K, Wosu C, Nieroda C, **Sardi A.** Port site metastases in patients with stage IV appendiceal neoplasm. Presented at SSO 65th Annual Symposium, Orlando, Florida, March 2012

Sardi A. Surgical Options: Management of Primary NETs in the presence of Metastases. Presented to the Neuroendocrine Tumor Regional Conference, Linthicum Heights, MD, April 20, 2012

Sardi A. Management of Ovarian Cancer with Peritoneal Metastases: This is how we do it. Presented at Workshop on The

Management of Peritoneal Metastases; Medstar Washington Hospital Center, Washington, D.C., June 21, 2012

Sardi A. Manejo de Carcinomatosis Peritoneal. Presented at XII Congreso Sociedad Dominicana De Hematologia Y Oncologia. Dominican Republic, September 6-9, 2012

Sardi A. Aspectos Tecnicos de la Cirugia Hepatica. Presented at XII Congreso Sociedad Dominicana De Hematologia Y Oncologia. Dominican Republic, September 6-9, 2012

Sardi A., V Gushchin, C Nieroda, M Sittig, S Shankar, J Francis, R MacDonald. Repeated Cytoreductive Surgery and Hyperthermic Intraperitoneal Chemotherapy (CRS/HIPEC) in Patients with Peritoneal Carcinomatosis from Appendiceal Cancer. Presented at the 8th International Workshop on Peritoneal Surface Malignancy, Berlin, Germany, October 30 – November 2, 2012

Sardi A. The evolution in the surgical management of breast cancer. Presented in Cali, Colombia, November 25, 2012.

B Gallagher, **A Sardi**, C Nieroda, H El-Halabi, V Gushchin. Incidental Papillary Carcinoma in Patients Treated Surgically for Benign Thyroid Disease. Poster Presentation at the Southeastern Surgical Congress 2013 Annual Scientific Meeting, Jacksonville, Florida, February 9-12, 2013

Sardi A, Gushchin V, Nieroda C, Sittig M, Shankar S, Francis, J, MacDonald R, Ledakis P. Melphalan: A Promising Agent in

Patients Undergoing Cytoredutive Surgery and Hyperthermic Intraperitoneal Chemotherapy (CRS/HIPEC). Poster presentation at the the 2013 Annual Cancer Symposium of the Society of Surgical Oncology

Suven Shankar MBBS, Michelle Sittig RN, Carol Nieroda MD, Ryan MacDonald PhD, Vadim Gushchin MD, **Armando Sardi MD.** The Role of Cytoreductive Surgery and Hyperthermic Intraperitoneal Chemotherapy in Patients with Primary Peritoneal Carcinoma with Failed Conventional Treatment. Poster presentation to the the 2013 Annual Cancer Symposium of the Society of Surgical Oncology

Suven Shankar MBBS, Michelle Sittig RN, Carol Nieroda MD, Ryan MacDonald PhD, Vadim Gushchin MD, **Armando Sardi MD.** Extended Survival in the Elderly Undergoing Cytoreductive Surgery/Hyperthermic Intraperitoneal Chemotherapy (CRS/HIPEC). Poster presentation at the 2013 Annual Cancer Symposium of the Society of Surgical Oncology

Sardi A, The Role of HIPEC in Rare Gynecological Malignancies. Presented at the 2 Day Medical Education Course with Live HIPEC Surgery at Mercy Medical Center, June 20-21, 2013.

Sardi A, Peritoneal Carcinomatosis: Not the End of the Road. Presented at the Oncology Grand Rounds at Monter Cancer Center, North Shore LIJ Health System, June 28, 2013.

TRAINING COURSES (Faculty)

Head and Neck Surgery review. Presented at the General Surgery Review Course of the Osler Institute as mock oral exam preparation with didactic lecture in New Orleans, Louisiana, February 22, 1991; in Pittsburgh, Pennsylvania, September 21, 1991; in Seattle, Washington, June 7, 1991; and in Jacksonville, Florida, December 14, 1991

Laparoscopic hernia repair. Panama City, Panama, July 23-25, 1992.

Laparoscopic hernia repair. Fundación Santa Fe, Bogota, Colombia, July 27, 1992.

Laparoscopic hernia repair. Universidad del Valle, Cali, Colombia, July 28, 1992 and August 6, 1992.

Cirugia laparoscopica su desarrollo y ultimos avances. XV Aniversario Fundacion, Hospital de Diagnostico, San Salvador, El Salvador, March 30- April 2, 1993.

Advanced laparoscopic techniques: colon resection, small bowel resection, highly selective vagotomy, adrenalectomy and splenectomy. Held at Hospital Universitario del Valle, Cali, Colombia; May 27-28, 1993.

Minimally invasive approach to solid organ surgery. Sponsored by The Minimally Invasive Surgical Training Institute (MISTI) Held at St. Joseph Medical Center, Baltimore, Maryland; August 1, 1997. Course Director.

Minimally invasive approach to solid organ surgery. Sponsored by The Minimally Invasive Surgical Training Institute (MISTI) Held at St. Joseph Medical Center, Baltimore, Maryland. September 29, 1997. Course Director.

Minimally invasive approach to solid organ surgery. Sponsored by the Minimally Invasive Surgical Training Institute (MISTI) Held at St. Joseph Medical Center, Baltimore, Maryland. February, 1998. Course Director.

Minimally invasive approach to solid organ surgery. Sponsored by the Minimally Invasive Surgical Training Institute (MISTI) Held at St. Joseph Medical Center, Baltimore, Maryland. June, 1998. Course Director.

Minimally invasive approach to solid organ surgery. Sponsored by the Minimally Invasive Surgical Training Institute (MISTI) Held at St. Joseph Medical Center, Baltimore, Maryland. September, 1998. Course Director.

Minimally Invasive Procedures for Breast Cancer, Melanoma, Hyperparathyroidism. Sponsored by the Clinical Research Center and Comprehensive Breast Center at St. Agnes HealthCare, Baltimore, Maryland. Nov. 9-10, 1998. Course Director.

Minimally Invasive Procedures for Breast Cancer, Melanoma, Hyperparathyroidism. Sponsored by the Clinical Research Center and Comprehensive Breast Center at St. Agnes HealthCare, Baltimore, Maryland. Jan 14-15, 1999. Course Director.

Minimally invasive approach to solid organ surgery. Sponsored by the Minimally Invasive Surgical Training Institute (MISTI) Held at St. Joseph Medical Center, Baltimore, Maryland. February 26, 1999. Course Director.

Minimally invasive approach to solid organ surgery. Sponsored by the Minimally Invasive Surgical Training Institute (MISTI) Held at St. Joseph Medical Center, Baltimore, Maryland. April 16, 1999. Course Director.

Minimally Invasive Procedures for Breast Cancer, Melanoma, Hyperparathyroidism. Sponsored by the Clinical Research Center and Comprehensive Breast Center at St. Agnes HealthCare, Baltimore, Maryland. April 22-23, 1999. Course Director.

Minimally invasive approach to solid organ surgery. Sponsored by the Minimally Invasive Surgical Training Institute (MISTI) Held at St. Joseph Medical Center, Baltimore, Maryland. June 14, 1999. Course Director.

Minimally Invasive Procedures for Breast Cancer, Melanoma, Hyperparathyroidism. Sponsored by the Clinical Research Center and Comprehensive Breast Center at St. Agnes HealthCare, Baltimore, Maryland. September 9-10, 1999. Course Director.

Sentinel Node Biopsy for Breast Cancer. Sponsored by the Department of Surgery of Northwest Hospital Center, Baltimore, Maryland. October 2, 1999. Course Faculty.

Minimally Invasive Techniques for Breast Care. Sponsored by the Clinical Research Center and Comprehensive Breast Center at St. Agnes HealthCare, Baltimore, Maryland. March 10, 2000. Course Director.

Minimally Invasive Techniques for Breast Care. Sponsored by the Clinical Research Center and Comprehensive Breast Center at St. Agnes HealthCare, Baltimore, Maryland. June 9, 2000. Course Director

Minimally Invasive Techniques for Breast Care. Sponsored by the Clinical Research Center and Comprehensive Breast Center at St. Agnes HealthCare, Baltimore, Maryland. November 17, 2000. Course Director

Minimally Invasive Techniques for Breast Care. Sponsored by the Clinical Research Center and Comprehensive Breast Center at St. Agnes HealthCare, Baltimore, Maryland. March 21, 2002. Course Director

Minimally Invasive Techniques for Breast Disease. Sponsored by the Clinical Research Center and Comprehensive Breast Center at St. Agnes HealthCare, Baltimore, Maryland. February 6, 2003. Course Director

SPECIAL COURSES
Breast Endoscopy and Intraductal Biopsy Training. Acrueity, Inc. December 2003

MammoSite Radiation Therapy System Clinical Training Program. April 24, 2004

Seven habits of highly effective management. Franklin Covey November 2005

Fundamentals of Capsule Endoscopy: Clinical Applications and Practice Integration. September 2007

Laparoscopic Liver Course – The University of Pittsburgh Liver Cancer Center – September 2006

Basic General Surgery - Lower Porcine Program "Da Vinci Training" – Philadelphia, PA May 2011

PUBLICATIONS/MANUSCRIPTS

Sardi A. Carcinoma del remanente gástrico: Una entidad clínica insidiosa. Colombia Medica 1986;17(4):214-7.

Sardi A, Singer J. Insulinoma and gastrinoma in Wermer's disease (MEN-1). Arch Surg.1987;122:835-6.

Sardi A, Gokli A, Singer J. Diverticular disease of the cecum and ascending colon: A review of 881 cases. Am Surg. 1987;53:41-5.

Sardi A, Parikh K, Singer J, Minken S. Mesenteric cysts. Am Surg. 1987;53:58-60.

Sardi A, Minken S. The placement of intracaval filters in an anomalous left-side vena cava. J Vasc Surg. 1987;6:84-6.

Sickle-Santanello B, O'Dwyer PJ, Mojzisik CM, Tuttle SE, Hinkle GH, Rousseau M, Schlom J,Thurston MO, Nieroda CA, **Sardi A**, Minton JP, Martin EW Jr. Radioimmunoguided surgery using the monoclonal antibody B72.3 in colorectal tumors. Dis Col Rect. 1987;30:761-5.

Sardi A, Minton JP, Nieroda CA, Sickle-Santanello BJ, Young D, Martin EW Jr. Multiple re-operations in recurrent colorectal carcinoma: An analysis of morbidity, mortality and survival. Cancer 1988; 61:1913-19.

Sardi A, Hinkle GH, Hill TL, Young D, Siddiqi MA, Agnone C, Martin EW Jr. Preferential prolonged binding to tumor enhances radioimmunolocalization of monoclonal antibodies. Internat J Biolog Markers. Pro Amer Assoc Cancer Res 1988;29:385.

Minton JP, Hamilton W, **Sardi A**, Nieroda CA, Sickle-Santanello BJ, O'Dwyer PJ. Results of surgical excision of one to thirteen hepatic metastases in 98 consecutive patients. Arch Surg. 1989;124:46-8.

Sardi A, Workman M, Mojzisik CM, Hinkle GH, Nieroda CA, Ferrara PJ, Agnone C, Farrar WB, Martin EW Jr. Intra-abdominal recurrence of colorectal cancer detected by radioimmunoguided surgery (RIGSTM). Arch Surg. 1989;124:55-9.

Nieroda CA, Mojzisik CM, **Sardi A**, Farrar W, Siddiqi MA, Ferrara PJ, James A, Thurston MOO, Martin EW Jr. Staging of carcinoma of the breast using a hand-held gamma detecting probe and monoclonal antibody B72.3. Surg Gynecol Obstet. 1989;169:35-40.

Sardi A, Minton JP, Mojzisik CM, Nieroda CA, Ferrara PJ, Thurston MO, Martin EW Jr. The use of a hand-held gamma detector improves the safety of isolated limb perfusion. J Surg Oncol. 1989;41:172-6.

Farrar WB, Nieroda CA, Scott M, **Sardi A**. Pancreatic heterotopia: Case report and literature review. Contemp Surg.1989; 35:25-9.

Nieroda CA, Siddiqi MA, Hinkle GH, Hill TL, Mojzisik CM, Olsen J, Rousseau M, Gersman M, Houchens D, **Sardi A**, Thurston MO, Martin EW Jr. An assessment of prolonged reactivity of seven monoclonal antibodies against CX-1 tumor xenografts using a novel hand-held gamma detecting probe. J Invest Surg. 1989; 2:227-0.

Sardi A, Siddiqi MA, Hinkle GH, Rousseau M, Gersman M, Hill TL, Olsen J, Tuttle SE, Young D, Houchens D, Thurston MO, Martin EW Jr. Localization by hand-held gamma detecting probe of tumor labeled with antibody 'cocktail'. J Surg Res. 1989;47(3):227-4.

Sardi A, Agnone C, Nieroda CA, Mojzisik CM, Hinkle GH, Ferrara P, Farrar WB, Bolton J, Thurston MO, Martin EW Jr. Radioimmunoguided surgery in recurrent colorectal cancer: The role of carcinoembryonic antigen, computerized tomography, and physical examination. So Med J. October 1989;82:1235-0.

Nieroda CA, Mojzisik CM, **Sardi A**, Ferrara PJ, Hinkle GH, Thurston MO, Martin EW Jr. The impact of radioimmunoguided surgery (RIGSTM) on surgical decision making in colorectal cancer. Dis Col Rect November, 1989;32(11):927-2.

Sardi A, Nieroda CA, Sickle-Santanello BJ, Minton JP, Martin E Jr. CEA-directed multiple surgical procedures for recurrent colon cancer confined to the liver. Am Surg 1990;56(4):255-9.

Sauter E, Bolton J, Willis G, Farr G, **Sardi A**. Improved survival after pulmonary resection of metastatic colorectal carcinoma. J Surg Oncol 1990;43:135-8.

Sauter E, **Sardi A**, Hollier L, Cooper E, Bolton J. Prognostic value of DNA flow cytometry in thymomas and thymic carcinomas. So Med J June, 1990;83(6);656-9

Sauter E, Vauthey J, **Sardi A**, Bolton J. Selective management of patients with neutropenic enterocolitis using peritoneal lavage. J Surg Oncol 1990;45:63-7.

Sardi A, Martucci J, Anderson G. In vitro study of implantable devices in the delivery of drugs: A word of caution. Reg Cancer Treatment, 1990; 3:228-1.

Risher W, **Sardi A**, Bolton J. Urachal abnormalities in Adults: The Ochsner Experience. So Med J September, 1990; 83(9):1036-9.

Nieroda CA, Mojzisik CM, Ferrara PJ, **Sardi A**, Hinkle GH, Thurston MO, Martin EW Jr. Radioimmunoguided surgery in primary colon cancer. Cancer Detect Prev 1990;14(6): 651-6.

Galloway J, **Sardi A**, DeConti R, Bolton J. Changing trends in thyroid surgery - 38 years' experience. The American Surgeon, January 1991; 57(1):18-0.

Cohen A, Martin E, Lavery I, Daly J, **Sardi A**, Aitken D, Bland K, Mojzisik CM, Hinkle GH. Radioimmunoguided surgery: A preliminary report of a multicenter trial to evaluate the use of the radiolabeled B72.3 monoclonal antibody in colorectal cancer. Arch of Surg. March 1991; 126(3):349-2.

Cohen A, Martin EW Jr, Lavery I, Daly J, **Sardi A**, Aitken D, Bland K, Mojzisik CM, Hinkle GH. Radioimmunoguided surgery using iodine B72.3 in patients with colorectal cancer. Arch Surg 1991;126:349-2.

Sardi A, Agnone C, Anderson M, Bolton J, Sundgaard-Riise K, Nieroda CA, Minton JP. Low-dose cyclophosphamide enhances helper-to-suppressor ratios. Cancer Detect Prev 1991; 15(3):217-4.

Sauter E, Hollier L, Bolton J, Ochsner J. **Sardi A**. The prognostic importance of DNA flow cytometry In parangliomas of the carotid body. J Surg Onc 1991;46(3):151-3.

Sardi A, Facundus E. A simplified aseptic technique to obtain large blood samples in the rat model. Lab Animal 1991;20(7):51-2

Risher W, **Sardi A**. Urachal abnormalities in the elderly: A case report. Surgical Rounds 1991; 14(7):618-0.

Sardi A, Walters P. A modified mandibular swing procedure for resection of carcinoma of the oropharynx. Head & Neck 1991; September/October, pp 394-7.

Sardi A, Eckholdt G, McKinnon W, Bolton J. The significance of mammographic findings following breast conserving therapy for carcinoma of the breast. Surg, Gyn & Obstet 1991; 173(4):309-2.

Nguyen J, McMullen K, **Sardi A**. Lobular carcinoma in situ within a fibroadenoma: A case report. J La State Med Soc 1991; 143(10)33-5

Bolton J, **Sardi A**, Merritt, C, Mitchell W. Ultrasound guided fine needle aspiration cytology with immunoperoxidase confirmation prior to reexploration for recurrent hyperparathyroidism. J La State Med Assn 1991; 143(10):37-1.

Sardi A, Agnone C, Pelligrini A. Renal metastases from papillary thyroid carcinoma. J La State Med Soc 1992; 144(9): 416-0.

Sardi A, Facundus E, McKinnon W, Skenderis B, Bolton J. Management of cancer of the opposite breast following breast preservation. Int Surg 1992; 77(4): 289-2.

Bolton J, **Sardi A**, Bowen J, Ellis JK. Transhiatal and transthoracic esophagectomy: A comparative study. J Surg Onc 1992; 51(4):249-3.

Sardi A, Bolton J, Mitchell W Jr., Merritt C. Immunoperoxidase confirmation of ultrasonic guided fine needle aspirates in patients with recurrent hyperparathyroidism. Surg Gyn Obstet 1992; 175(6):563-8.

Ferguson E, **Sardi A**, Beckman E. Spontaneous rupture of splenic hamartoma: A case report. J La State Med Soc 1993; 145(2):48-2.

Kuske R, Farr G, Harris K, Bolton J, **Sardi A**, McKinnon W, Kardinal C, Cole J, Pickett T, Graham M, Fineberg B. Is Breast Preservation Possible in Women with Large, Locally Advanced Breast Cancers? J La St Med Soc 1993; 145(4):165-7.

Sardi A, McKinnon W. Laparascopic Adrenalectomy for Primary Aldosteronism. JAMA 1993; 269(8):989-0.

Sardi A. Colostomy isolation during abdominal surgery. Intl Surg 1993; 78(2):146-7.

Sardi A, McKinnon WM. Laparascopic Adrenalectomy for Primary Aldosteronism. Surg Lap & Endos., 1994; 4(2): 86-1.

Sardi A, Bolton JS, Hicks TC, Skenderis BS. Total Pelvic Exenteration With or Without Sacral Resection in Patients with Recurrent Colorectal Cancer. So Med J.1994; 87:363-9.

Sardi A. Laparascopic Splenectomy for Patients with Thrombocytopenic Purpura. Surg Lap & Endos 1994; 4(4): 316-9.

Urban J, **Sardi A,**Colandrea J,. Solid and Papillary Epithelial Neoplasm Diagnosis and Treatment: A Case Study. MMJ 1995;44:699-2.

Metzger N, **Sardi A**, Lawrence G. Laparascopic adrenalectomy in a patient with Cushing Syndrome. MMJ 1996; 45:407-0.

Singh K, **Sardi A**, Conaway G, Spiegler E. Gamma detecting probe and isosulphan blue for localization of sentinel node in malignant melanoma. MMJ 1996;46:476-1.

Sardi A, Akbarov A, Conaway G. Management of primary and metastatic tumors to the liver. Oncology 1996. 10(6):911-25.

Pergolizzi J, **Sardi A,**, Pelczar M, Conaway G. Merkle cell carcinoma: An aggressive malignancy. Am Surg. 1997; 63:450-4.

Irwin JF, **Sardi A**, Waterfield W, Poussin H: Multi modality treatment in the management of esophageal cancer: Neoadjuvant chemo-radiotherapy followed by transhiatal esophagectomy. MMJ 1997; 46: 471-6.

Ehrmantraut W, **Sardi A**. Laparascopic assisted small bowel resection. Am Surg. 1997; 63:996-001.

Eckholdt G, **Sardi A**. The surgical approach to the octogenarian with gastrointestinal malignancy. Surg Rounds.1998; 21(6):287-94.

Moran J, **Sardi A**, Singer J. Retrosternal Goiter: A six-year institutional review. Am Surg. 1998; 64(9):889.

McLean R, **Sardi A**. Gastric cancer: An overview with emphasis on early gastric cancer. MMJ. August 1998; 47(4):191.

Stancofski E, **Sardi A**. Conaway G. Successful outcome in Swan Ganz catheter induced rupture of pulmonary artery. Am Surg 1998; 64(11):1062-5

Sardi A, Ojeda H. Laparoscopic Resection of a Benign True Cyst of the Spleen with the Harmonic Scalpel Producing High Levels of CA 19-9 and Carcinoembryonic Antigen (CEA). Am Surg. December, 1998; 64(12):1149-4.

Pergolizzi J, Auster M, Conaway G, **Sardi A**. Cryosurgery for unresectable primary hepatocellular carcinoma: a case report and review of literature. Am Surg. May 1999; 65(5):402-5.

Singer J, **Sardi A**, Conaway G, Spiegler E. Minimally invasive parathyroidectomy utilizing a gamma detecting probe intraoperatively. MMJ. March/April 1999:55-8.

Sardi A, Rehman S, Speigler E, Colandrea J, Frishberg D. Sentinel Lymph node mapping for staging breast cancer:

Preliminary results of a prospective study. MMJ. May/June 1999; 48(3):105-0.

Sardi A, Ojeda H, Barco, E. Cryosurgery: adjuvant treatment at the time of resection of a pelvic recurrence in rectal cancer. Am Surg. November 1999;65(11):1088-1

Stone M, Sardi A, Conaway, G, Rehman S. Hepatic Resection at a Community Hospital. J Gastrointestinal Surg. 2000;4:349-4

McMasters KM, Wong SL, Tuttle TM, Carlson DJ, Brown C, Noyes RD, Glaser R, Vennekotter DJ, Turk PS, Tate PS, Sardi A, Edwards M. Preoperative lymphoscintigraphy for breast cancer does not improve the ability to accurately identify axillary sentinel lymph nodes. Ann Surg. 2000 May;231(5):724-1

Cervone A, Sardi A, Conaway G. Intraoperative ultrasound (IOUS) is essential in the management of metastatic liver lesions. Am Surg. July 2000;66(7):611-5

Ojeda H, Sardi A, Totoonchie A. Sarcoidosis of the Breast: Implications for the General Surgeon. Am Surg. December 2000;66(12):1144-8

Martin R, McMasters KM, Edwards MJ, Wong SL, TuttleT, Carlson DJ, Tate PS, Brown C, Noyes RD, Glaser R, Vennekotter DJ, Turk PS, Sardi A, Cerrito P. Practical guidelines for optimal gamma probe detection of sentinel lymph nodes in breast cancer: Results of a multi-institutional study. Surgery. 2000 August;128(2):139-4

McMasters KM, Tuttle TM, Carlson DJ, Brown C, Noyes RD, Glaser R, Vennekotter DJ, Turk PS, Tate PS, **Sardi A**, Cerrito P, Edwards M. Sentinel-lymph-node biopsy for breast cancer. A suitable alternative to routine axillary dissection in multi-institutional practice when optimal technique is used. J Clin Oncol. 2000 Jul;18(13):2560-6

Heeringa B., **Sardi A.** Bleeding hepatic adenoma; expectant treatment to limit the extent of liver resection. Am Surg. October 2001;67: 927-9

Sardi A, Rehman S, Spiegler E, Colandrea J, Frishberg D, Singh H, Regan P, Totoonchie A, Merchant D, Hochuli S, Setya V. The benefit of using two techniques for sentinel lymph node mapping in breast cancer. Am Surg. 2002;68(1): 24-8

Sher Ahmed A; Buscema J; **Sardi A.** A case report of recurrent epithelial ovarian cancer metastatic to the sternum, diaphragm, costae, and bowel managed by aggressive secondary cytoreductive surgery without postoperative chemotherapy" Gynecol Oncol. 2002;86:91-4

Averbach A, Akbarov A, Sidel T, Mech K, Parandian B, Waterfield W, Poussin-Ropsillo H, Chang D, **Sardi A**. Results of curative therapy for esophageal cancer in a community training hospital. Int Surg. 2002 January-March;87(1):31-7

Ganti Al, Gordon J. **Sardi A.** Laparoscopic treatment of large cysts of the liver and spleen is ineffective. Am Surg. 2002 Nov;68(11):1012-7

Parisky YR, **Sardi A**, Hamm R, Hughes K, Esserman L, Rust S, Callahan K. Efficacy of computerized infrared imaging analysis in the discrimination of mammographically suspicious lesions. Am J Roentgenol. 2003 Jan; 180(1): 263-9

Krishnaiah G, Sher-Ahmed A, Ugwu-Dike M, Regan P, Singer J, Totoonchie A, Spiegler E, **Sardi A.** Technetium-99M sestamibi scintimmamography complements mammography in the detection of breast cancer. Breast J. 2003 Jul-Aug;9(4): 288-4

Del Carmen MG, Hughes KS, Halpern E, Rafferty E, Kopans D, Parisky YR, **Sardi A**, Esserman L, Rust S, Michaelson J. Racial differences in mammographic breast density. Cancer. 2003 Aug 1; 98(3):590-6

Gann M, **Sardi A**, Bieligk S. Improved results using ultrasound guidance for central venous access. Am Surg. 2003; 12:1104-7

Peterson RM. **Sardi A.** Hemicorporectomy for chronic pressure ulcer carcinoma: 7 years of follow up. Am Surg. 2004 June; 70 (6): 507-1

Karpinski S, **Sardi A.** Thorascopic Resection of Mediastinal Intrathymic Parathyroid Adenoma: A case Report. Am Surg. 2005 Dec; 71:1070-2

Stephenson S, Mech K, **Sardi A**. Lung Cancer Screening with Low-Dose Spiral Computed Tomography. Am Surg. 2005 December; 71(12):1015-7

Sneed D, Hamdalah I, **Sardi A.** Absence of the Retrohepatic Inferior Vena Cava-What the surgeon should know. Am Surg. 2005 June;71(6):502-4

Peterson, R, **Sardi A**, Ballo M. Analytic Uncertainty and Clinical Impact of Human Growth Factor Receptor-2 (HER-2/neu) testing in a Community Hospital. Surgical Rounds 2006, July; 281-283

Esquivel J, Sticca R, Sugarbaker P, Levine E, Yan T D, **Sardi A**, et al. Cytoreductive Surgery and Hyperthermic Intraperitoneal Chemotherapy in the Management of Peritoneal Surface Malignancies of Colonic Origin: A Concensus Statement. Ann Surg Oncol 2006. DOI: 10.1245/s10434-006-9185-7

Semino-Mora C, Liu H, McAvoy T, Nieroda CA, Studeman K, **Sardi A**, Dubois A. Pseudomyxoma Peritonei: Is disease progression related to microbial agents? A Study of Bacteria, MUC2 and MUC5AC Expression in Disseminated Peritoneal Adenomucinosis and Peritoneal Mucinous Carcinomatosis. Ann Surg Onc. 2008 May;15(5):1414-23.

Gushchin V, Ross A, Miller D, Nieroda CA, Kalesan B, Studeman K, Kostuik P, **Sardi A**. Complete Cytoreduction Offers Long-term Survival in Patients with Peritoneal Carcinomatosis from Appendiceal Tumors of Unfavorable Histology. JACS. 2009Sept; 2009(3): 308-312

Ross A, **Sardi A**, Nieroda CA, Merriman B, Gushchin V. Clinical Utility Of Elevated Tumor Markers In Patients With Disseminated

Appendiceal Malignancies Treated By Cytoreductive Surgery And HIPEC European Journal of Surgical Oncology 36 (2010) pp. 772-776

Esquivel J, Chua TC, Stojadinovic A, Melero JT, Levine EA, Gutman M, Howard R, Piso P, Nissan A, Gomez-Portilla A, Gonzalez-Bayon L, Gonzalez-Moreno S, Shen P, Stewart JH, Sugarbaker PH, Barone RM, Hoefer R, Morris DL, **Sardi A**, Sticca RP. Accuracy and clinical relevance of computed tomography scan interpretation of peritoneal cancer index in colorectal cancer peritoneal carcinomatosis: A multi-institutional study. J Surg Oncol. 2010 Nov 1;102(6): 565-70

El Halabi H, Gushchin V, Francis J, Athas N, MacDonald R, Nieroda C, Studeman K, **Sardi A.** The role of cytoreductive surgery and heated intraperitoneal chemotherapy (CRS/HIPEC) in patients with high-grade appendiceal cancer and extensive disease. Ann Surg Oncol (2012) 19:110-114

El Halabi H, Gushchin V, Francis J, MacDonald R, Athas N, **Sardi A.** Prognostic Significance of Lymph Node Metastases in Patients with High-grade Appendiceal Cancer. Ann Surg Oncol (2012) 19:122-125

El Halabi H, Ledakis P, Francis J, Athas N, MacDonald R., Studeman K, Wosu C, Nieroda C, Gushchin V, **Sardi A.** The Role of Systemic Chemotherapy in Patients Undergoing Cytoreductive Surgery and Heated Intraperitoneal Chemotherapy for Carcinomatosis from Appendiceal Cancer. Submitted to J Surg Oncol. Oct. 2011

El Halabi H, **Sardi A**, MacDonald R, Studeman K, Francis J, Nieroda V, Gushchin V. Delay of Cytoreductive Surgery and Heated Intraperitoneal Chemotherapy (CRS/HIPEC) in Patients with Appendiceal Neoplasm. Submitted to Am Surg Jan 2012

1Chua T, 2Moran B, 3Sugarbaker P, 4Levine E, 5Glehen O, 5Gilly F, 6Baratti D, 6Deraco M, 7Elias D, **8Sardi A**, 1Liauw W, 3Yan T, 9Barrios P, 10Gómez Portilla A, 11de Hingh I, 12Ceelen W, 13 Pelz J, 14Piso P, 15González-Moreno S, 16Van Der Speeten K, 1Morris D. Early and Long-term Outcome Data on 2298 Patients with Pseudomyxoma Peritonei of Appendiceal Origin Treated by a Strategy of Cytoreductive Surgery and Hyperthermic Intraperitoneal Chemotherapy. JCO July 2012 30(20)2449-56

Turaga K, Levine E, Barone R, Sticca R, Petrelli N, Lambert L, Nash G, Morse M, Abdel-Misih R, Alexander HR, Attiyeh F, Bartlett D, Bastidas A, Blazer T, Chu Q, Chung K, Dominquez-Parra L, Espat NJ, Foster J, Fournier K, Garcia R, Goodman M, Hanna N, Harrison L, Hoefer R, Holtzman M, Kane J, Labow D, Li B, Lowy A, Mansfield P, Ong E, Pameijer C, Pingpank J, Quinones M, Royal R, Salti G, **Sardi A**, Shen P, Skitzki J, Spellman J, Stewart J, Esquivel J. Consensus Guidelines from The American Society of Peritoneal Surface Malignancies on Standardizing the Delivery of Hyperthermic Intraperitoneal Chemotherapy (HIPEC) in Colorectal Cancer Patients in the United States. Ann Surg Oncol 2013 June 21; DOI 10.1245/ s10434-013-3061-z

PUBLISHED ABSTRACTS

Nieroda CA, Farrar WB, Mojzisik CM, **Sardi A**, Siddiqi M, Tuttle J, Martin EW Jr. Radioimmunoguided surgery: The intra-operative detection of tumor in breast cancer patients. In: Breast cancer research and treatment, William J. McGuire, M.D., ed. - Martinus Nijhoff Publishers. October 1987;10:86

Sardi A, Hinkle GH, Hill TL, Young D, Siddiqi MA, Agnone C, Martin EW Jr. Preferential prolonged binding to tumor enhances radioimmunolocalization of monoclonal antibodies. Proc Am Assoc Cancer Res 1988;29:285

Sardi A, Agnone C, Mojzisik CM, Farrar WB, Hinkle GH, Ferrara PJ, Nieroda CA, Bolton J, Thurston MO, Martin EW Jr. Radioimmunoguided surgery in recurrent colorectal cancer: The role of CEA, CAT scan and physical examination. So Med J 1988;81(9):10

Sardi A, Agnone C, Anderson G, Bolton J, Sundgaard-Riise K, Nieroda CA, Minton JP. Low-dose cyclophosphamide enhances helper-to-non-helper ratios. Cancer Detect Prev 1989;14(1):121

Nieroda CA, Mojzisik CM, **Sardi A**, Ferrara PJ, Hinkle GH, Thurston MO, Martin EW Jr. Radioimmunoguided surgery in primary colon cancer. Cancer Detect Prev 1989;14(1):151

Nieroda CA, Agnone C, **Sardi A**, Houchens D, Hinkle GH, Bondo S, Martin EW Jr. Comparison of biokinetics of first and second generation monoclonal antibodies. Am. Assoc. Cancer Res., 1989;30(#1428):360

Sauter E, Bolton J, Willis G, Farr G, **Sardi A**. Improved survival after pulmonary resection of metastatic colorectal carcinoma. So Med J 1989;82:40

Risher W, **Sardi A**, Bolton J. Urachal abnormalities in adults: The Ochsner experience. So Med J 1989;82:97

Sauter E, Hackney J, Bolton J, Hollier L, **Sardi A**. Prognostic value of DNA flow cytometry in thymomas and thymic carcinomas. So Med J 1989;82:8

Sardi A, Eckholdt G, McKinnon W, Bolton J. Management of cancer of the opposite breast following breast preservation. J Cancer Res Clin Oncol (Part I) 1990; 116;199. Intl Surg 1992;1:262

Bolton J, Kuske R, **Sardi A**, McKinnon W, Hawkins R, Scroggins T. Radiation Therapy (RT) in Early Stage Breast Cancer: Can Brachytherapy Replace External Beam Whole Breast Radiation Therapy (WhBRT) in Patients Treated with Breast Conserving Therapy (BCT) - Results of a Pilot Study. Proc Am Soc Cl Onc, 148:1993

Sardi A, Kunjummen B, Rehman S, Spiegler E, Colandrea J, Frishberg D, Singh H, Regan P, Totoonchie A, Merchant D. The impact of using two techniques in SLN mapping for breast cancer. European Journal of Surgical Oncology 2000; 26:262

Sardi A Hamdallah I. Diagnostic Value of Preoperative FNA in Follicular and Hurthle Cell Neoplasms. Ann Surg Oncol. 2005;12(2)176:93

Semino-Mora C, **Sardi A**, Liu H, McAvoy T, Dubois A. Pseudomyxoma Peritonei: An Infectious disease? Ann Surg Oncol. February 2006;13(2)172: 83-84

Franco, G., Kostuik, P, Nieroda, C., Cianos, R., Merriman, B. **Sardi A.** Impact of Cytoreductive Surgery and Hyperthermic Intraperitoneal Chemotherapy in Patients with Disseminated Intra-abdominal Carcinomatosis. Ann Surg Oncol. February 2006;13(2)185: 87

Baraki Y, Kostuik P, Merriman B, Nieroda CA, **Sardi A**. Long term survival following cytoreductive surgery and intraperitoneal hyperthermic chemotherapy for disseminated appendiceal tumors. J Clin Oncol. June 2006, 24(18S)4128:209s

Sardi A, Thillainathan V, Nieroda CA, Merriman B, Kostuik P. Comparison of open and closed techniques of delivery of hyperthermic chemotherapy following cytoreductive surgery in patients with peritoneal carcinomatosis. J Clin Oncol. June 2006; 24(18S)14067:629s

Munalula J, Nieroda CA, Kostuik P, Holter D, Kalesan B, Gushchin V, **Sardi A**. Cytoreductive surgery followed with intraperitoneal hyperthermic chemotherapy in elder patients with appendiceal carcinomatosis. Ann Surg Oncol. February 2007;14(2)254:109

Gushchin V, Ross A, Nieroda CA, Kalesan B, Kostuik P, Holter D, **Sardi A**. Common tumor markers predict extent of disease and success of cytoreductive surgery in patients with appendiceal malignancies. J *Clin Oncol* 26: 2008, May 2008; 15527

Sardi A, Omohwo C, Nieroda C, Holter D, Athas N, Gushchin V. Bowel Complications In Patients with Peritoneal Carcinomatosis of Appendiceal Origen Treated with Cytoreductive Surgery and Hyperthermic Intraperitoneal Chemotherapy. Ann Surg Oncol. February 2010;17(1)165: 85-86

Thieme H, Gushchin V, **Sardi A,** Athas N. Peritoneal Carcinomatosis in the Geriatric Patient: Outcomes with Cytoreductive Surgery and HIPEC. Ann Surg Oncol. February 2010;17(1) 290: 123

El Halabi H, Gushchin V, Francis J, MacDonald R, Athas N, **Sardi A.** Lymph node metastasis predicts survival in patients with high-grade appendix cancer. Ann Surg Oncol. February 2011; 18(1) 154: 86

El Halabi H, Gushchin V, Francis J, MacDonald R, **Sardi A.** Patients with high-grade appendix cancer and extensive disease benefit from cytoreductive surgery and heated intraperitoneal chemotherapy. Ann Surg Oncol, February 2011; 18(1) 203: 101

El Halabi H, Gushchin V, Francis J, Nieroda C, **Sardi A.** The role of cytoreductive surgery in patients with carcinomatosis from high-grade appendix cancer in the era of modern systemic chemotherapy. J Clin Oncol 29: 2011 (suppl; abst 4080)

Chua T, Moran B, Sugarbaker P, Levine E, Glehen O, Gilly F, Baratti D, Deraco M, Elias D, **Sardi A**, Liauw W, Yan T, Barrios P, Gómez Portilla A, de Hingh I,Ceelen W, Pelz J, Piso P, González-Moreno S, Van Der Speeten K, Morris D. Early and Long-term Outcome Data on 2298 Patients with Pseudomyxoma Peritonei of Appendiceal Origin Treated by a Strategy of Cytoreductive Surgery and Hyperthermic Intraperitoneal Chemotherapy. J Clin Oncol 30, 2012 (suppl 4; abstr 532)

A Sardi, V Gushchin, C Nieroda, M Sittig, S Shankar, J Francis, R MacDonald, P Ledakis. Intraperitoneal Melphalan in Patients Undergoing Cytoredutive Surgery and Hyperthermic Intraperitoneal Chemotherapy (CRS/HIPEC). Poster presentation at the 8th International Workshop on Peritoneal Surface Malignancy, Berlin, Germany, October 30 – November 2, 2012

RECENTLY SUBMITTED ABSTRACTS
Wosu C, El-Halabi, Wong M, Gallagher B, Francis J, Studeman K, Ledakis P, Nieroda C, Gushchin V, **Sardi A**. Progression of Peritoneal Adenomucinosis to the Scrotum: A Rare Occurrence Treated with Cytoreductive Surgery and Hyperthermic Intraperitoneal Chemotherapy. Accepted for presentation at the Seventh International Symposium on Regional Cancer Therapies, February 2012, Florida

Wosu C, El-Halabi, Wong M, Gallagher B, Francis J, Studeman K, Ledakis P, Nieroda C, Gushchin V, **Sardi A**. The Role of Cytoreductive Surgery and Hyperthermic Intraperitoneal Chemotherapy in Patients with Primary Peritoneal Carcinoma.

Submitted for presentation to Society for gynecologic Oncology
Feb 2012 Winter Meeting

Wosu C, El-Halabi, Wong M, Gallagher B, Francis J, Studeman
K, Ledakis P, Nieroda C, Gushchin V, **Sardi A.** Cytoreductive
Surgery and Hyperthermic Intraperitoneal Chemotherapy in the
Management of High Grade Uterine Sarcomas with Peritoneal
Dissemination. Submitted for presentation to Society for gyne-
cologic Oncology Feb 2012 Winter Meeting.

El Halabi H, Gushchin V, Francis J, MacDonald R, Studeman
K, Wosu C, Nieroda C, **Sardi A.** Port site metastases in patients with stage IV appendiceal neoplasm. Accepted by SSO
for poster presentation at 65th Annual Symposium, March 2012,
Orlando, Florida

Gilbreath J, Semino-Mora C, Friedline C, Liu H, Bodi K, McAvoy
T, Francis J, Nieroda C, **Sardi A**, Dubois A, Lazinski D, Camilli
A, Testerman T, Merrell D.S. A Core Mictobiome Associated with
the Peritoneal Tumors of Pseudomyxoma Peritonei. *Accepted for
Publication by Orphanet Journal of Rare Disease*

BOOK CHAPTERS
Minton JP, **Sardi A**. Carcinomambryonic antigen and second-
look operation. Problems in General Surgery; January-March
1987;4(1):104-114.

Nieroda CA, **Sardi A**, Martin EW Jr. CEA-directed second-look
surgery. In: Current Surgical Therapy-3 Ed: Cameron J. Pg. 155-
161. B.C. Decker Inc.: Philadelphia, PA, 1989.

Sardi A, Minton JP, Chevinsky A. Multiple operations for recurrent colorectal cancer. Sem in Surg Oncol, 1991;7:146-156.

Sardi, A., Hollier L. Bilateral laparoscopic lumbar sympathectomy. In: Ascer E. Hollier LH, Strandness Jr DE, etal: Haimovici's Vascular Surgery, Principals and Techniques. Fourth edition. Blackwell Science Incorporated 1996. 86;pp 1134-1136.

Sardi, A. Tratamiento del Carcinoma *In-Situ* de la Mama. pp 533-542 In: Actualización en Cirugía del Aparato Digestivo, Vol. VIII, 2nd edition. Ed: Jarpyo, S.A. 1996.

Sardi, A. Técnica de Recesión del Intestino Delgado por Laparoscopia Asistida. In: Actualización en Cirugía del Aparato Digestivo, pp 273-276 Vol. VIII, 2nd edition. Ed: Jarpyo, S.A. 1996.

Sardi, A. Tratamiento del Cáncer Gástrico en 1994. In: Actualización en Cirugía del Aparato Digestivo, pp 321-333 Vol. VIII, 2nd edition. Ed: Jarpyo, S.A. 1996.

Sardi, A. Problemas Especiales Durante Colicestectomía Laparoscópica. In: Actualización en Cirugía del Aparato Digestivo, pp 201-207 Vol. IX, 2nd edition. Ed: Jarpyo, S.A. 1996.

Sardi, A. Adrenalectomía por Laparoscopia: Técnica Quirúrgica. In: Actualización en Cirugía del Aparato Digestivo, pp 281-285 Vol. IX, 2nd edition. Ed: Jarpyo, S.A. 1996.

Sardi, A. Manejo Quirúrgico del Cancer Recurrente del Colon y Recto. pp 353-367 In:: Actualización en Cirugía del Aparato Digestivo, Vol. IX, 2nd edition. Ed: Jarpyo, S.A.1996.

Sardi, A, Aggressive Surgical Management of Metastatic Colorectal Cancer to the Liver Coping November/December 1997, 43-44

Sardi, A., Hollier L. Bilateral laparoscopic lumbar sympathectomy. In: Ascer E. Hollier LH, Strandness Jr DE, etal: Haimovici's Vascular Surgery, Principals and Techniques. Fifth edition. Blackwell Science Incorporated 2003. Chapter 55; pp 657-659

Sardi A, El-Halabi H, Gushchin V, Shankar S. Neoplasms of the appendix. Published in Hem/Onc Clinics Journal. September 2012

VIDEOS

RADIOIMMUNOGUIDED SURGERY. Martin EW Jr, Nieroda CA, **Sardi A**, Lange M. 41st Annual Meeting of the Southwestern Surgical Congress, April 23-26, 1989, Monterey, California.

THE USE OF RADIOIMMUNOGUIDED SURGERY IN RESECTING RETROPERITONEAL RECURRENT COLORECTAL CANCER. **Sardi A**, Martin EW Jr. Presented at the 1989 Annual Meeting of the Society of Surgical Oncology, May 21-24, 1989, San Francisco, CA; Presented at the American College of Surgeons 1989 Clinical Congress, Oct 15-20, 1989 Atlanta, GA; and the American College of Surgeons Medical Motion Picture Library. Presented at the 1992 Clinical Congress

Workshop Session of the American College of Surgeons, October 12, 1992. Held in the Motion Picture Library of the American College of Surgery.

A MODIFIED MANDIBULAR SWING PROCEDURE FOR RESECTION OF CARCINOMA OF THE OROPHARYNX. **Sardi A**, Walters P. Presented at the 36th Annual Meeting of the Society of Head and Neck Surgeons, May 20-22, 1990, Washington D.C.; Presented at the 1990 Clinical Congress of the American College of Surgeons, October 7-12, San Francisco, CA.

ISOLATED HYPERTHERMIC PERFUSION IN THE MANAGEMENT OF METASTATIC COLON CANCER. **Sardi A**, Hayes D.

SISSON PROCEDURE FOR RESECTION OF CARCINOMA OF THE THYROID. **Sardi A**, Skenderis B. Presented at the annual meeting of the Society of Head and Neck Surgeons, May 1-4, 1991, Maui, HI; presented at to the 1991 Annual Meeting of the American College of Surgeons, October 20-25, 1991, Chicago, IL. Presented at the 1992 Annual Meeting of the International College of Surgeons. Presented at (Greater Baltimore Medical Center). Held in the motion picture library of the American College of Surgeons. Third Annual Darrell A. Jacques Symposium.

THE MANDIBULAR SWING PROCEDURE FOR RESECTION OF CARCINOMA OF THE TONGUE. **Sardi A**, Smith D. 1991.

LAPAROSCOPIC HERNIA REPAIR. **Sardi A**. Presented at Panama City, Panama, July 23-25, 1992; also presented at Fundación Santa Fe, Bogota, Colombia, July 27, 1992; also presented at Universidad del Valle, Cali, Colombia, July 28, 1992.

LAPAROSCOPIC SPLENECTOMY FOR A PATIENT WITH IDIOPATHIC THROMBOCYTOPENIC PURPURA. **Sardi, A**. Presented at the Society of Surgical Oncology meeting, Los Angeles, CA, March 18-21, 1993. Presented at the Joint Meeting of the Surgical Association of Louisiana and the Louisiana Chapter of the American College of Surgeons, January 23-24, 1993, New Orleans, LA. Presented at the 2nd Congress of Private Hospitals of Guatemala, March 11-13, 1993, Guatemala City, Guatemala. Presented at Laparoscopic Procedures course at Hospital Universitario del Valle, Cali, Colombia, May 28, 1993. Presented at XVII Congreso Nacional de Cirugía; Cuenca, Ecuador, May 25-26, 1993. Presented at the 4th World Congress International and Joint Meeting of Surgery, Gastroenterology and Endoscopy, Madrid, Spain, October 27-30, 1993. Held in the Motion Picture Library of the American College of Surgeons.

LAPAROSCOPIC ASSISTED SMALL BOWEL RESECTION. **Sardi, A**. Presented at Laparoscopic Procedures course held at Hospital Universitario del Valle, Cali, Colombia; May 25-26, 1993. Presented at XVII International Meeting of Surgery, Madrid, Spain, May 1994.

LAPAROSCOPIC POSTERIOR TRUNCAL VAGOTOMY AND ANTERIOR HIGHLY SELECTIVE VAGOTOMY. **Sardi A**. Presented at Laparoscopic Procedures course held at Hospital

Universitario del Valle, Cali, Colombia; May 28, 1993. Presented at XVII International Meeting of Surgery, Madrid, Spain, May 1994.

LAPAROSCOPIC RIGHT ADRENALECTOMY IN A PATIENT WITH ALDOSTERONOMA. **Sardi A**, McKinnon WMP. Presented at Laparoscopic Procedures course held at Hospital Universitario del Valle, Cali, Colombia; May 28, 1993. Presented at XVII International Meeting of Surgery, Madrid, Spain, May 1994.

LAPAROSCOPIC LEFT ADRENALECTOMY FOR PRIMARY ALDOSTERONISM. **Sardi A**, McKinnon WMP. Presented at Laparoscopic Procedures course to be held at Hospital Universitario del Valle, Cali, Colombia; May 28, 1993. Presented at the 1993 Clinical Congress of the American College of Surgeons, San Francisco, CA, October 10-15, 1993. Presented at the 4th World Congress International and Joint Meeting of Surgery, Gastroenterology and Endoscopy, Madrid, Spain, October 27-30, 1993. Presented at XVII International Meeting of Surgery, Madrid, Spain, May 1994. Held in the Motion Picture Library of the American College of Surgeons

RADICAL NEPHRECTOMY AND PARTIAL RESECTION OF THE VENA CAVA WITH EXTRACTION OF TUMOR THROMBUS IN RENAL CELL CARCINOMA. **Sardi, A**. Presented at the 1993 Clinical Congress of the American College of Surgeons, San Francisco, CA, October 10-15, 1993. Held in the Motion Picture Library of the American College of Surgeons.

BILATERAL LAPAROSCOPIC LUMBAR SYMPATHECTO-MY. **Sardi A**, Hollier LH. Presented at the Motion Picture exhibition of the American College of Surgeons. Chicago, October 7-12, 1994.

HEMICORPORECTOMY IN A PATIENT WITH SQUAMOUS CELL CARCINOMA ARISING FROM A SACRAL DECUBITUS ULCER (MARJOLIN'S ULCER). **Sardi A**. Presented at the 83rd Annual Clinical Congress of the American College of Surgeons, Chicago, Illinois, October, 1997. Held in the Motion Picture Library of the American College of Surgeons.

LAPAROSCOPIC TREATMENT OF A TRUE CYST OF THE SPLEEN PRODUCING HIGH LEVELS OF CEA AND CA 19-9. **Sardi A**, Ojeda, H. Presented at the American College of Surgeons 1998 Clinical Congress Meeting, Orlando, Florida, October 26, 1998. Held in the Motion Picture Library of the American College of Surgeons.

LAPAROSCOPIC RIGHT ADRENALECTOMY FOR PHEOCHROMOCYTOMA **Sardi A**, Submitted for presentation at the Southeastern Surgical Congress, Lake Buena Vista, Florida, February 2000.

ULTRASOUND GUIDED PLACEMENT OF CENTRAL VENOUS ACCESS DEVICES. **Sardi A.** Submitted to the Annual Congress of the American College of Surgeons. New Orleans, 2004. Held in the Motion Picture library of the American College of Congress.

INVITED COMMENTARIES

Sardi A, Aggressive Surgical Management of Metastatic Colorectal Cancer to the Liver. Coping. November/December 1997, 43-44.

JOURNAL REVIEW

Sardi A, Guest Reviewer for The Annals of Thoracic Surgery

Sardi A, Guest Review for Colombia Médica

GRANT SUPPORT

Herbert J. Block Memorial Fund - Surgical Oncology Research Fund. Sardi A, Minton JP. Toxicity of cyclophosphamide and its effects on the lymphocyte populations in the rat. June 1987-July 1988.

MRDF, The Ohio State University. Sardi A, Nieroda CA, Minton JP. Highly purified recombinant human Interleukin-2 in the treatment of minimal residual metastatic carcinoma to the liver in the rat. June 1, 1987-May 21, 1988.

American Cancer Society, Inc., Ohio Division. Sardi A, Minton JP. Evaluation of Interleukin-2 and cyclophosphamide in the treatment of minimal residual disease metastatic to the liver. July 1, 1987-June 30, 1988.

MRDF, The Ohio State University. Sardi A, Siddiqi MAA, Nieroda CA, Martin EW Jr. Determination of ischemic intestine by the NeoprobeTM portable radioisotope detector. August 1, 1987-July 31, 1988.

Phase I-II Clinical Study: The intraoperative detection of colorectal cancer by radiolabeled B72.3 monoclonal antibody. Multicenter trial -**Sardi A**, Principal Investigator.

Alton Oschner Foundation Medical Research Fund. **Sardi, A**. Interleukin-2 and 5-Fluorouracil in the treatment of metastatic adenocarcinoma to the liver in the rat.

Alton Ochsner Medical Foundation Research Fund. **Sardi A**. Somatostatin analogue SMS 201-995 in the treatment of metastatic colon carcinoma to the liver in the rat.

Sardi A. A multicenter clinical study using a technetium-labeled monoclonal antibody to evaluate the mediastinum in newly diagnosed non-small cell lung cancer.

Alton Ochsner Medical Foundation Research Fund. **Sardi A**. HER-2 neu, ras, and myconcogene in human adenocarcinomas.

Phase III clinical study: Intraoperative detection of I B72.3 monoclonal antibody in patients with colorectal cancer - multicenter trial - **Sardi A**., Principal Investigator.

Sardi A, Witherspoon L, Bolton J, Timmcke A, Hicks T, Ray J, Gathright G. ^{111}In-CYT-103 as a diagnostic imaging agent in the management of patients with colorectal denocarcinoma. 1990 -1993.

Kline R, **Sardi A**, Witherspoon L. Intravenously administered ^{111}In-CYT-103 in the imaging of ovarian cancer. 1990 - 1993.

Sardi A, Bolton JS, Witherspoon L, Timmcke AE, Hicks TC. Administration of Repeat Intravenous Doses of ^{111}In-CYT-103 in the Detection of Recurrent Colorectal Carcinoma. 1990 - 1993.

Sardi A, Bolton J, Witherspoon L, Timmcke A, Hicks T, Ray J, Hathright G. Dose-Range Efficacy and Safety of Intravenously Administered ^{111}In-CYT-372 in the Imaging of Colorectal Carcinoma. 1990 - 1993.

Sardi A, Bolton J, Witherspoon L, Timmcke A, Hicks T, Ray J, Gathright J. Intravenously Administered ^{99m}Tc-CYT-380 in the Detection of Colorectal Carcinoma. 1990 - 1993.

Sardi A, Bardot S, Witherspoon L, Bodie B, Weed W, Fuselier H. Administration of Intravenous Doses of ^{111}In-CYT-356 in the Detection of Occult Prostrate Carcinoma. 1990 - 1993.

Sardi A, Bardot S, Witherspoon L, Bodie B, Weed W, Fuselier H. Multicenter Study of Intravenously Administered ^{111}In-CYT-356 in the Evaluation of Patients with Primary Prostrate Cancer prior to Staging Pelvic Lymph Node Dissection. 1990 - 1993.

Sardi A, Bolton J, Hicks T, Farr G, Witherspoon L, Opelka F, Timmcke A, Gathright J, Landry K. Comparative Study of the Efficacy and Safety of Intravenously Administered ^{111}In-CYT-103 (^{111}In-satumomab pendetide) and ^{111}In-CYT-372, Given Individually and in Combination, for the Detection of Colorectal Carcinoma. 1990 - 1993.

Sardi A, Witherspoon L, Bolton J, Hicks T, Timmcke A, Gathright G, Landry K. Phase II Clinical Study: The Intraoperative Detection of Colon and Rectal Cancer using the CC49 Monoclonal Antibody in Patients with a Prior Exposure to Murine Monoclonal Antibody. 1990 - 1993.

Sardi A, Hicks T, Witherspoon L, Bolton J, Timmcke A, Gathright J, Opelka F, Farr G, Landry K. Phase III Clinical Study: The comparison of current diagnostic modalities to the radioimmunoguided surgery™ (RIGS®) system using 125I CC49 monoclonal antibody for patients with primary adenocarcinoma of the colon and rectum.

Sardi A, Gralla , Witherspoon L, McFadden P, Bolton J, Onofrio J, Shuler S, Landry K. A Multicenter Clinical Study Using a Technetium-Labeled Monoclonal Antibody for Imaging Patient with Small Cell Lung Cancer.

Sardi A, McFadden P, Van Meter C, Witherspoon L, Bolton J, Onofrio J, Gralla R, Emory W, Shuler S, Burns C, Farr G, Landry K. A Multicenter Clinical Study to Compare Imaging of Non-Small Cell Lung Cancer with a Technetium-Labeled Monoclonal Antibody Produced by Two Different Manufacturers.

Sardi A, Spiegler E, Pelczar M, Roffe M, Merchant D, Totoonchie A, Colandrea J, Zalucki J, Signor W, Setya V, Singer J, Conaway G. A Phase III Clinical Study: The Comparison of Current Diagnostic Modalities to the Radioimmunoguided Surgery (RIGS) System using 125I CC49 Monoclonal Antibody for Patients with Intraabdominal Metastatic Adenocarcinoma of the Colon and Rectum. 1994 - 1996.

Sardi A, Spiegler E, Pelczar M, Roffe M, Merchant D, Totoonchie A, Colandrea J, Zalucki J, Signor W, Setya V, Singer J, Conaway G. Phase III Clinical Study: The Comparison of Current Diagnostic Modalities to the Radioimmunoguided Surgery (RIGS) System using 125I CC49 Monoclonal Antibody for Patients with Primary Adenocarcinoma of the Colon and Rectum. 1994 - 1996.

Sardi A, Spiegler E, Pelczar M, Conaway G. Radioimmunos-cintigraphy of Occult Colorectal Carcinoma with OncoSpect (99mTc-88BV59) a Totally Human Monoclonal Antibody Multicenter Study. 1995 - 1997.

Sardi A, Spiegler E, Pelczar M, Conaway G. Radioimmunos-cintigraphy of Recurrent/Metastatic Colorectal Carcinoma with OncoSpect (99mTc-88BV59) a Totally Human Monoclonal Antibody Multicenter Study. 1995 - 1997.

Sardi A, Spiegler E, Pelczar M, Conaway G. Radioimmunos-cintigraphy of Colorectal Carcinoma after Repeat Infusion with OncoSpect (99mTc-88BV59) a Totally Human Monoclonal Antibody Multicenter Study. 1995 - 1997.

Sardi, Spiegler E, Pelczar M, Conaway G. A Multi-center Evaluation of OncoSPECT CR/Colorectal (^{99m}Tc-88BV59H21-2V67-66) in the Detection of Extrahepatic Metastases in Colorectal Cancer Patients. 1995 - 1997.

Sardi A, Spiegler E, Pelczar, Roffe M, Conaway G. Phase II Clinical Study: The Intraoperative Detection of Colon and Rectal Cancer Using CC49 Monoclonal Antibody in Patients With a Prior Exposure to Murine Monoclonal Antibody. 1995-1997

Buscema J, **Sardi A**, Spiegler E, Conaway G. Radioimmunoscintigraphy with ^{99m}Tc-88BV59 in Patients with Suspected Ovarian Cancer. 1996 - 1997.

Sardi A, Spiegler E, Gormley P, Mech K, Minken S, Pelczar M, Waterfield W, Conaway G. Phase I/II Study of Radioimmunoscintigraphy with 'X' (Technetium Tc^{99m} Labeled Human Monoclonal Antibody Votumumab) in Patients with Suspected Non-Small Cell Lung Cancer. 1997-1999.

Sardi A, Spiegler E, Frishberg D, Waterfield W, Ottaviano Y, Gormley P, Griffiths D, Conaway G. Sunbelt Melanoma Trial (SMT): Multicenter Trial of Adjuvant Interferon Alfa-2b for Melanoma Patients with Early Lymph Node Metastasis Detected by Lymphatic Mapping and Sentinel Lymph Node Biopsy. 1997.

Sardi A, Spiegler E, Conaway G, Brice J. Protocol 9707: Immunoscintigraphy of Colorectal Cancer with Technetium Tc^{99m} Labeled Human Monoclonal Antibody "X" 1998-2000.

Sardi A, Chen A, Sladek G, Ottaviano Y, Waterfield W, Pelczar M, Conaway G, et al. A Phase I (CAP) with Detox™ PC in adult Patients with Adenocarcinomas of the Gastrointestinal Tract, Breast, Lung. 1997-1998.

Sardi A, Spiegler E, Totoonchie A, Setya V, Singer J, Signor W, Falcao K, Mercnat D, Parikh K, Meyer G, Hochuli S, Gheba M, Conaway G, Parce P, Regan P. Technetium 99m Sestamibi (Miraluma Tm) Scintimammography in the detection of occult breast cancer 2000-2001.

Sardi A, Singh R, Singer J, Signor W, Falcao K, Hochuli S, Merchant D, Totoonchie A, Setya V, Hayward G, Parikh K, Meyer G, Gheba M, Regan, P, White R, Hazlinsky N. Clinical study of the Examination of Breasts for the Identification of Suspicious Tissue using Clinical Examination and Mammography with and without computerized Thermal Imaging System (CTI). 1999-2001

Sardi A, Meyer G, Regan P. A Study of the IsoMed™ Pump Model 8472 for the Hepatic Arterial Infusion of Chemotherapy. 2000

Sardi A, Falcao K, Gheba M, Gormley P, Griffiths D, Meyer GM, Sarshar A, Setya V, Singer J, Totoonchie A, Waterfield W, Zalucki J, Regan P, Flack J. A Non-Randomized Multi-Center Phase I/II Study Of Active Specific Immunotherapy In Patients With Stage II and Stage III Colon Cancer 2001.

Sardi A. Susan G. Komen Breast Cancer Foundation grant to increase minority accrual for STAR trial 2001-2002.

Sardi A. Susan G. Komen Breast Cancer Foundation Grant "Shining Stars: Breaking down barriers to Hispanic and African

American Women Participation in Breast Cancer Clinical Trials"
May 2002-2003

Sardi A, Zalucki J, Cain M, Regan P, Conaway G, Parce P. A Multicenter Phase III, Double-Blind, Placebo-Controlled, Parallel Study of ADL 8-2698 in Opioid-Induced Postoperative Bowel Dysfunction/Postoperative Ileus. 2002

Sardi A A Phase III Randomized Double-Blind Pivotal Trial of Immunotherapy with BCG plus a Polyvalent Melanoma Vaccine, *CancerVax®* versus BCG plus a Placebo as a Post-Surgical Treatment for Stage III Melanoma. 2002 to 2005.

Sardi A A Phase III Randomized Double-Blind Trial of Immunotherapy with Vaccine, *CancerVax®* plus BCG versus Placebo plus BCG as a Post-Surgical Treatment for Stage IV Melanoma. 2002-2005

Sardi A, Death P. A Phase III Study of Heat Shock Protein-Peptide Complex (HSPPC-96) versus Physician's Choice Including Interleukin-2 and/or Dacarbazine/Temozolomide-Based Therapy and/or Complete Tumor Resection in Stage IV Melanoma. (Completed)

Sardi A. A ProspectiveStudy of The Prognostic Significance of Microsatellite Instability in Patients with Early Age-of-Onset Colorectal Cancer. (Protocol Z0190 – ACOSOG).

Sardi A. A Phase III Randomized Double-blind Study of Adjuvant STI571 (GleevecTM) Versus Placebo in Patients

Following the Resection of Primary Gastrointestinal Stromal Tumors (GIST). 2003 to present.

Sardi A Identification of Tumor-Associated Surface Proteins, Including Glycoproteins, in Various Cancer Specimens: A Search for Novel Therapeutic Targets. 2003 to 2006.

Sardi A. Vishwanathan K. JHH/Ductal Lavage in high-risk patients. 2004 to 2006.

Sardi A. Intraductal Approach to breast cancer. Ductoscopy Mammary in patients with nipple discharge. 2004 to 2006

Sardi A. Phase III Randomized Double-blind study of Adjuvant ST1571 (Gleevec TM) Versus placebo in patients following the resection of primary gastrointestinal stromal Tumors (GIST) 2005

Sardi A. Identification of tumor-associated surface proteins including Glycoproteins in various cancer specimens: A Search for Novel Therapeutic Targets. 2005

Sardi A. Vishwanathan K. JHH/Ductal Lavage in high-risk patients. 2005

Sardi A. A Phase II Study of Radiofrequency Ablation of Unresectable Liver Tumors with Hepatic Artery Infusion Chemotherapy. 2006

Sardi A. A Prospective Study of The Prognostic Significance of Microsatellite Instability in patients with early age-of-onset Colorectal Cancer (Protocol Z0190-ACOSOG) 2006

Sardi A. Phase 3 Clinical Trial to Evaluate the Safety and Efficacy of Treatment with 2 mg Intralesional Allovectin-7® Compared to Dacarbazine (DTIC) or Temozolomide (TMZ) in Subjects with Recurrent Metastatic Melanoma. 2008 to 2010

CURRENT PROJECTS
Sardi A Hyperthermic Intraoperative Intraperitoneal Chemotherapy for Intraabdominally Advanced Colorectal, Appendix, gastric, small bowel, primary peritoneal, Ovarian Cancers, Peritoneal Mesothelioma and Sarcomas. This is a prospective database of Dr. Sardi's and Mercy Medical Center's HIPEC patients treated for intraabdominally advanced cancers from 1994 to present. This database yields significant analytical data to refine future treatment protocols and enhance patient care. 1994 to present

Sardi A. Mercy Medical Center "Pilot Study" to Demonstrate the Link between H. Pylori and Development of Pseudomyxoma Peritonei (PMP). This study involves the evaluation of scientific data obtained from blood and tissue samples removed during cytoreductive surgery to determine the presence of various enteric bacteria (including H. Pylori). It further investigates the effects of antibiotics administered both pre and post surgery on the growth rate and recurrence of these tumors as well as patient survival. 2006 to present

Sardi A. Multi-center Selective Lymphadenectomy for Melanoma Trial II: A Phase III Multi-center Randomized Trial of Sentinel Lymphadenectomy and Complete Lymph Node Dissection versus Sentinel Lymphadenectomy Alone in Cutaneous Melanoma Patients with Molecular or Histopathological Evidence of Metastases in the Sentinel Node. 2006 to present

Sardi A. Chemofx assay as a predictor of outcome in patients who have peritoneal carcinomatosis treated with cytoreductive surgery, intraperitoneal hyperthermic chemotherapy (IPHC) with Mitomycin C, with or without post IPHC chemotherapy. The assessment of the effectiveness of multiple chemotherapy agents on tumor tissue removed during cytoreductive surgery identifies the optimal chemotherapy agent most suited to effectively treat these cancerous tumors. 2007 to present

Sardi A. International PM Registry 2010. A world-wide, multi-institutional retrospective database creating the largest available dataset for a comparative study of conventional treatment versus radical cytoreduction with IP therapy for mucinous appendiceal cancer. This international registry is used for univariate and multivariate analysis of factors associated with survival. 2010 to present

Sardi A. A Study of Tissue Molecular Markers and Their Relationship to Treatment and Outcome in Appendiceal Cancer with Pseudomyxoma Peritonei (PMP). The objectives of this research are to determine the expression or mutations in the genes K-ras, EGFR, B-RAF, VEGF, ERCC1, HER 2/Neu, TS, as well as the status of MSI in tumor tissue from advanced appendiceal cancer and to study a potential association between those genes and tumor grade, and treatment outcome such as time to recurrence, overall and disease free survival after cytoreductive surgery with hyperthermic intraperitoneal chemotherapy and systemic chemotherapy. 2010 to present

Doctor Armando Sardi's current curriculum vitae can be found on the Mercy Hospital, Baltimore, website, http://www.mdmercy.com/centerExcellence/cancer_services/surgical_oncology/sardi_cv.html.

Endnotes

One

[1]Sporn, M. B. 1996. The war on cancer. *The Lancet* 347:1377–1381.

[2]Carole Langrall also maintains three blogs, one to help others with Conn's disease and two that feature exquisite photography (http://www.hyperaldo-steronism.blogspot.com, http://www.internationalflowerspy.blogspot.com, and http://www.neglectedbeauty.blogspot.com). See also Carole Langrall's "Medical Mystery," as told to Beth Howard, *Harmony Magazine* January–February 2011.

[3]Hippocrates actually used two related terms, *carcinos* and *carcinoma* to describe nonulcer-forming and ulcer-forming tumors. Almost surely best known for his Hippocratic oath, variations of which are still in use today, he has a very interesting life story. Prior to Hippocrates, medicine was commingled with religion and philosophy, and he was one of several in his time who wanted to turn it into a hard science and ultimately a profession. Such heresy was punished with a twenty-year prison sentence, during which time he wrote *The Complicated Body*, among other works.

[4]Edwin Smith was an American Egyptologist who allegedly purchased the papyrus from an Egyptian dealer named Mustapha Aga in 1862. There have been two translations of this seventeen-page document, one of which is by James Henry Breasted, with the technical help of Dr. Arno B. Luckhardt (Breasted, J. H. 1930. *The Edwin Smith Surgical Papyrus: Published in Facsimile and Hieroglyphic Transliteration with Translation and Commentary in Two Volumes.* Chicago: University of Chicago Press.) Page 463 contains the possible reference to breast cancer.

[5]Suessmann, M. Moses ben Maimon. *Encyclopaedia Judaica*, second edition. (2003).

[6]Celsus, A. C. 1935. *On Medicine, Book V*, published in vol. II of the Loeb Classical Library edition.

[7]Mukherjee, S. 2010. *The Emperor of All Maladies*. New York: Scribner, 44.

[8] Paget, S. March 1889. The distribution of secondary growths in cancer of the breast. *The Lancet* 133(3421):23. Incidentally Paget also asserts in this work that the idea was partly inspired by a German man named Fuchs, who wrote *"Das Sarkom des Uvealtractus"* (1882) in *Graefe's Archiv für*

Opthalmologie, XII, 233. Fuchs used terms that have been translated as "embolus" and *"recipient tissue."*

[9]Dr. John Singer's wife Ruth began her career as a health official in Carroll County, Maryland, then moved on to become the director of local health for the entire state. After her retirement, she joined the Chase Brexton clinic, which at the time only served AIDS patients but began to expand its services several years later. She passed away in 2013.

[10]http://www.youtube.com/watch?v=0BImHu1LXyA&feature=related. There was a certain urgency to Matt Blastowich's case, which occurred in 2003 or 2004. Dr. Sardi went through with the operation even though the patient's insurance claim was denied. Sardi believes the insurance company eventually decided to pay, but he's not sure. Those records would now be at St. Agnes Hospital in Baltimore. As of fall 2012, Mr. Blastowich was still doing quite well.

[11]http://www.youtube.com/watch?v=bV7qpRGYWls.

[12]At a 2011 oncology seminar, Dr. Sardi, speaking of a surgery after which the cancer recurred, remarked, "We must have missed something." Dr. Sugarbaker replied, "I'm not sure you missed anything, Armando. I just think that perhaps the concept that microscopic disease should always be eradicated by HIPEC doesn't always come true. You might have done the cytoreduction down to CC00 [lower than the lowest score] and still have this sort of situation one year later." Sugarbaker also noted, "We need a better HIPEC."

[13]Sardi continued, "There are hundreds and hundreds of publications in [peer-reviewed] medical journals showing the benefit of this approach for a variety of tumors. While there is not a single publication on chemotherapy alone showing one patient with peritoneal carcinomatosis—that means cancer all over the abdomen—that has been shown to be alive free of disease at five years. Well, there are many studies from several institutions that do this procedure showing its benefit with many patients alive beyond five years having a great quality of life and [a] cure from their cancer. We have a patient now living over eighteen years after she was told to go home and die." He added, "Let's start by saying that the survival rate free of cancer at five years is zero without this treatment...If you take a patient to this surgery with appendix cancer, for example—and there are different categories of appendix cancer—if you take the low grade, eighty percent will be cured. We're talking about alive, free of disease at five years. If you take the higher grades and intermediate grades, it is somewhere between thirty and fifty percent who will actually be free of disease in five years. If you talk about other cancers, for example, mesothelioma, and especially what we call the epithelial type,

the survival rate is close to eighty percent as well, [compared to] zero percent by chemotherapy alone." Interview with Armando Sardi, February 5, 2010.

[14]The following are the various acronyms for HIPEC, some of which are still in use: IPHP (intraperitoneal hyperthermic perfusion), HIIC (heated intra-operative intraperitoneal chemotherapy), IHCP (intraperitoneal hyperthermic chemoperfusion), IIC (intraoperative intraperitoneal chemotherapy, which may not have been heated initially), IPPC (intraperitoneal postoperative che-motherapy, not heated but with the suggestion that hyperthermia might im-prove results), IPCH (intraperitoneal chemohyperthermia) IPHC (intraperi-toneal hyperthermic chemotherapy), CHPP (chemohyperthermic peritoneal perfusion), IPRC (intraperitoneal regional chemotherapy), and HAPP (intra-peritoneal hyperthermic antiblastic therapy).

[15]The matter of precision in choosing the right temperature is not trivial. Oddly enough, one clear explanation of the topic, assuming the film has not been doctored in any way, comes from a commercial video that explains the capabilities of the Thermotron RF-8, a product developed by Yamamoto, a Chinese firm. In vitro, or observed in a test tube (as opposed to in vivo, ob-served in a live organism), the body's normal temperature is about 37° C, but noticeable disruption of the ability of cancer cells to divide doesn't kick much in until 42° C. Cancer-cell division apparently stops completely at 44° C. See the following video, http://www.youtube.com/watch?v=FbEiuXGVA3Q, minutes 1:06 to 4:16. The latest word on this subject appears to be Pelz, J. O. et al. Hyperthermic intraperitoneal chemotherapy in patients with peritoneal carcinomatosis: role of heat shock proteins and dissecting effects of hyper-thermia. *Annals of Surgical Oncology* 4:1105–13, doi:10.1245/s10434-012-2784–6, Epub March 2, 2013.

[16]Esquivel, J. Technology of hyperthermic intraperitoneal chemotherapy in the United States, Europe, China, Japan, and Korea. *Cancer Journal* 3:249–54. (2009).

[17]The very first clinical trial is often attributed to Daniel of Judah in 600 BC, who compared a vegetarian diet to the royal Babylonian diet over a ten-day period. (Stolberg, H. O., G. Norman, and I. Trop, Randomized controlled tri-als. *American Journal of Roentgenology,* July 2, 2004.

[18]Hill, A. B. The clinical trial. *New England Journal of Medicine* 247:113–119. (1952).

[19]Davis, D. 2007. *The Secret History of the War on Cancer*. New York: Basic Books, 325. Eddy went on to develop the Archimedes Model, proprietary software that can simulate real-life trials; at least in one instance, it simulated

a thirty-year trial in thirty minutes. See John Carey's article "Trimming Health Care Costs without Reforming the System," *Businessweek*, October 1, 2009. I don't know how Eddy's system works, or even whether it works, but it generally takes a decade for a drug to go from conception to FDA approval, with expenses that could be in the hundreds of millions of dollars, as it was for the monoclonal antibody herceptin, developed by Genentech for the treatment of certain breast cancers.

[20]Guidelines were established in 1947, in what is now referred to as the Nuremburg Code, as Nazi doctors had performed horrifying procedures and experiments, including the dissection of live patients. The Nuremburg Code was not law in the United States, but a civil suit clarified the necessity of informed consent when a certain plaintiff, Martin Salgo, underwent what he believed was a routine procedure, only to wake up paralyzed from the waist down. See Salgo v. Leland Stanford etc. Bd. Trustees, 154 Cal.App.2d 560 [Civ. No. 17045. First Dist., Div. One. Oct. 22, 1957]. The guidelines for informed consent were expanded in the early 1960s. A respected researcher, Chester Southam, began injecting people with cancerous cells in 1954, beginning with people who already had cancer, then moving on to healthy volunteers from a prison population and later to hospital patients. When, in 1963, he asked that patients in the Jewish Chronic Disease Hospital in Brooklyn be injected without their consent, three doctors refused, and when the injections were given anyway, these doctors resigned. They also sent their resignation letter to the press, which got the attention of New York State Attorney General Louis Lefkowitz. In the ensuing hearing, part of Southam's defense was that the practice of proceeding without consent, informed or otherwise, was widespread. The New York State Medical Grievance Committee found Southam and hospital director Emanuel Mandel guilty of "fraud or deceit and unprofessional conduct in the practice of medicine." The National Institutes of Health, which funded Southam, found that only nine of fifty-two of its funded institutions had any such informed-consent policy in place and rewrote the rules, stipulating that funding was contingent upon following them. (See also chapter seventeen in Rebecca Skloot's 2010 book *The Immortal Life of Henrietta Lacks*.)

[21] In the United States, for example, oversight is conducted at the federal level through the Office for Human Research Protections (OHRP) and the FDA, which requires an application for the use of any investigational new drug (IND). The study itself will have its own institutional review board (IRB), referred to as an "ethics committee" overseas. Large Phase II and Phase III trials also have a Data Safety Monitoring Board (DSMB), which is composed of a statistician and a group of scientists completely independent of the study itself. The DSMB has the power to shut down a trial at any time, which does

happen, though infrequently. The Department of Veterans Affairs (VA) has an additional set of rules to protect veterans. See Tomasz M. Beer, MD, and Larry W. Axmaker, EdD's 2012 book *Cancer Clinical Trials*, 93–96.

[22]Ibid, xvii.

[23] See Shah, S. Body hunting: the outsourcing of drug trials. *The Globalist*, January 31, 2007; Barlett, D. L. and J. B. Steele. Deadly medicine. *Vanity Fair*, January 2011; and Hearn, K. Unregulated clinical trials, exploitation and profit: how the FDA allows big pharma to exploit the poor in South America. *The Nation*, September 28, 2011.

[24]Phase I trials can begin once a new drug has been tested on two species. The primary purpose is to determine the safe dosage, though effectiveness can be monitored as well. The process also can be extremely time consuming as patients begin at a very low dose and work up from there. Phase Ø studies have been with us for less than a decade and involve a very small number of people for one or two weeks. They were designed to cut down on the costs and failure rate of Phase I trials. Phase IV studies are further studies of drugs already approved in the Phase III process. They often measure effectiveness and side effects over a longer period, as well as new applications for a drug.

[25]After two years 88 percent of the IHCP group was alive compared to 76 percent of the surgery-alone group; after four years, 76 percent to 58 percent and after eight years, 62 percent to 49 percent. See Fujimoto S. et al. Successful intraperitoneal hyperthermic chemoperfusion for the prevention of postoperative peritoneal recurrence in patients with advanced gastric carcinoma. *Cancer* 85:3, 529–34. (1999).

[26]Verwaal, V. J. et al. 8-year follow-up of randomized trial: cytoreduction and hyperthermic ontraperitoneal chemotherapy versus systemic chemotherapy in patients with peritoneal carcinomatosis of colorectal cancer. *Annals of Surgical Oncology* 9:2426–32, Epub June 3, 2008. For the first results, see Verwaal, V. J. et al. Randomized trial of cytoreduction and hyperthermic intraperitoneal chemotherapy versus systemic chemotherapy and palliative surgery in patients with peritoneal carcinomatosis of colorectal cancer. *Journal of Clinical Oncology* 21(20):3737–43. (2003).

[27]Elias, D. et al. Pseuomyxoma peritonei: a French multicenter study of 301 patients treated with cytoreductive surgery and intraperitoneal chemotherapy. *European Journal of Surgical Oncology* 36(5):456–62. Epub March 12, 2010. Part of the conclusion reads, "This large multicentric retrospective study confirms that cytoreductive surgery combined with PIC (with use of

hyperthermia) should be considered the gold standard treatment of PMP and should be performed in specialized centers."

Yan, T. D. and D. L. Morris. Cytoreductive surgery and perioperative intraperitoneal chemotherapy for isolated colorectal peritoneal carcinomatosis: experimental therapy or standard of care? *Annals of Surgery* 248(5):829–35. (2008).

Smeenk, R. M. et al. Survival analysis of pseudomyxoma peritonei patients treated by cytoreductive surgery and hyperthermic intraperitoneal chemotherapy. *Annals of Surgery* 245(1):104–109. (2007).

[28]Smith, G. C. S. and J. P. Pell. Parachute use to prevent death and major trauma related to gravitational challenge: systematic review of randomised controlled trials. *British Medical Journal* 327:20–27. (2003).

[29]Gómez, P. A. et al. The European contribution to "Sugarbaker's protocol" for the treatment of colorectal peritoneal carcinomatosis. *Revista Espanola de Enfermedades Digestivas* 101(2):97–106. (2009). Also see Nagarajan, P. et al. Sugarbaker procedure for pseudomyxoma peritonei. *Cochrane Database of Systematic Reviews,* iss. 1, article CD005659. (2006).

[30]These remarks were made at the 2009 Mesothelioma Symposium. At the time Sugarbaker compared seven studies on the results of traditional treatment of mesothelioma carcinoma compiled from 1988 to 1999. The median survival period ranged from nine months to fifteen months. In four hundred patients with mesothelioma carcinoma who had been treated with cytoreductive surgery and HIPEC, the median survival period was five years. See http://www.youtube.com/watch?v=fgHrIuox3pc (minutes 7:30–9:24).

[31]Davis, D., 2007, 285.

Two

[1]The snare works by lassoing the entire polyp then cutting it off at the base. See http://www.youtube.com/watch?v=p9a6oE-VJDA (minutes 1:38 to 2:34).

[2]Sugarbaker, P., as told to Bond, T. The evolution of treatment for peritoneal metastases. *Colorectal Cancer* 2(3):189–192. (2013).

[3]Paget, S. March 1889, 23.

[4]Moore, C. H. On the influence of inadequate operations on the theory of cancer. *Medico-Chirurgical Transactions* 50:245, 277. (1867).

[5]The most reliable places to find the cancer that had spread within the peritoneum were the greater omentum, the largest peritoneal fold, which covers the small intestines and transverse colon; the liver surface; the large bowel surface; and the cul-de-sac of Douglas, an area between the rectum and uterus in the female body. Also likely are the surface of the small bowel and the retroperitoneum, the peritoneal space behind the organs.

[6]Hanahan, D. and R. A. Weinberg, The hallmarks of cancer. *Cell* 100:57–70. (2000).

[7]Foulds, L. The experimental study of tumor progression: a review. *Cancer Research* 14:5, 327–339. (1954). Another important contributor to the observation of carcinogenesis was American pathologist Oscar Auerbach, who did a study comparing lung specimens of 1,522 smokers and nonsmokers. See Auerbach, O. and A.P. Stout. The role of carcinogens, especially those in cigarette smoke, in the production of precancerous lesions. *Proceedings of the National Cancer Conference 4*, 297-304. (1960). The earliest observations might possibly be attributed to the Greek-born American émigré Georgios Papanikolaou, most famous for his development of the Pap smear, designed to detect cancer cells in their earliest stages (sometimes referred to as precancer). Probably about thirty years passed between his first observations and his decision to express what he had found in terms of carcinogenesis.

[8]Hayflick, L. and Moorhead P. S. The serial cultivation of human diploid cell strains. *Experimental Cell Research* 25(3):585–621. (1961). Hayflick originally estimated that cells divide between forty and sixty times. The revised figure comes from Hanahan and Weinberg's article.

[9]Also of interest in Skloot's book is her portraiture of the descendants of Henrietta Lacks. It is obvious that she showed courage at various times to get the story.

[10]See Kolata, G. New view sees breast cancer as three diseases. *The New York Times*, April 1, 1997. Also see Bartlett, B. Mammograms: women face uncertainty—and cancer. *The [Louisville and Southern Indiana] Courier-Journal*, March 31, 2002.

[11]Spratt, J. S. et al. Hyperthermic peritoneal perfusion system in canines. *Cancer Research* 40:253–260. Spratt, J. S. et al. Clinical delivery system for intraperitoneal hyperthermic chemotherapy. *Cancer Research* 40:256–260. (1980). The use of hyperthermia in the treatment of cancerous limbs may have been first reported in 1967. See Cavaliere, R. et al. Selective heat sensitivity of cancer cells: biological and clinical studies. *Cancer* 20(9):1351–1381.

[12]Sugarbaker, P. H. Peritonectomy procedures. *Annals of Surgery* 221:1, 29–42. (1995).

[13]Heat alone can kill cancer cells without damaging normal cells. "Treatment at temperatures between 40° and 44° C is cytotoxic for cells in an environment with a low pO_2 and low pH, conditions that are found specifically within tumour tissue due to insufficient blood perfusion" (Van der Zee, J. Heating the patient: a promising approach? *Annals of Oncology* 13:1173–1184). (2002). When new chemo agents docetaxel, paclitaxel, iriotecan, oxaliplatin, and gemcitabine were tested, the enhanced cytotoxicity varied considerably. See Mohamed, F. et al. Thermal enhancement of new chemotherapeutic agents at moderate hyperthermia. *Annals of Surgical Oncology* 10(4):463–8. (2003). See also Esquivel, J. Technology of hyperthermic intraperitoneal chemotherapy in the United States, Europe, China, Japan, and Korea. *Cancer Journal* 15(3):249–54.

[14]According to Jennifer Francis, Mercy practice manager, when the patient is diagnosed and a treatment is recommended, the insurance company is called, and an authorization is given by the nurse or layperson receiving the call. If the insurance company does not have a standard policy for approving the treatment, the next step is a peer-to-peer review; for Francis this would mean having Dr. Sardi talk to a physician at the insurance company. If this didn't do the trick, Francis could then make a case in writing and include several recent peer-reviewed articles on the treatment. At this point she would be out of ammo, so to speak, and outside help would then be recommended, such as someone like Laurie Todd. Todd would not be constrained by certain HIPAA provisions; she could, for example, find a case in which the insurance company already had approved the treatment for a previous patient who'd had the same diagnosis and use that example in a further appeal. Another complication arises from the fact that many relatively small HMOs insist on keeping treatment within their network, but the network may not have a HIPEC practitioner or may have one with less experience than the patient is comfortable with.

[15]Todd, L. 2007. *Fight Your Health Insurer and Win*. Kirkland, WA: Healthwise Publications, 33–34.

[16]The original article can be found at Kusamura, S. et al. The importance of the learning curve and surveillance of surgical performance in peritoneal surface malignancy programs. *Surgical Oncology Clinics of North America* 21(4):559–76, doi:10.1016/j.soc.2012.07.011. Later, members of the same group concluded, "Surgical tutoring could *substantially* shorten the steep LC associated with CRS and HIPEC...Other factors that could influence the length of learning process should be identified." See Kusamura, S. et al.

Learning curve for cytoreductive surgery and hyperthermic intraperitoneal chemotherapy in peritoneal surface malignancies: analysis of two centres. *Journal of Surgical Oncology* 107(4):312–9, doi:10.1002/jso.23231, Epub August 23, 2012.

[17]In a 2011 international survey, two women with appendiceal cancer successfully delivered their babies prior to cytoreductive surgery and HIPEC. Seven women both conceived and successfully delivered a child after cytoreductive surgery and HIPEC, and another woman who had undergone oocytes retrieval and embryo cryopreservation [collecting eggs and then preserving embryos at subzero temperatures] prior to surgery birthed twins via a surrogate mother. Dr. Armando Sardi also has mentioned that some couples choose adoption. Ortega-Deballon, P. et al. Childbearing after hyperthermic intraperitoneal chemotherapy: results from an international survey. *Annals of Surgical Oncology* 18(8):2297–2301, doi:10.1245/s10434-0 11-1595-5. (2011).

[18]Todd, L. 2007, 35–36.

[19]DNA profiling—also called gene typing, DNA testing, and genetic fingerprinting—is a technique pioneered by Sir Alec Jeffreys and first reported in 1984. It is probably best known for identifying paternity and is also used in criminal cases. In medicine it is an option available to patients because, although more than 99 percent of DNA is the same from individual to individual, there are specific gene markers that are associated with certain diseases, such as breast cancer. The tests received considerable publicity in 2013 after actress and humanitarian Angelina Jolie took them and decided to undergo a preventative double mastectomy.

Three

[1]Safety procedures surrounding cytoreductive surgery and HIPEC have evolved over the years, and the current practice of walking the first day and up to four times every day thereafter is a case in point. Also, Venodyne, a sequential leg-compression device, is placed on the lower legs until the patient is walking regularly. In addition a blood thinner is administered daily during the postoperative period.

[2]McAuley's inheritance consisted of income streams but not a great deal of cash. She received income from the sale or lease of houses around Dublin, four annuities, the Coolock house in which she lived, Wide Street certificates, and dividends from a share in Apothecary Hall, a medical practice. The $2.7 million estimate is greatly dependent on the calculators available at http://www.measuringworth.com. See also Mary C. Sullivan's 2012 book *The Path of Mercy: The Life of Catherine McAuley*.

[3]http://www.cnn.com/video/?/video/health/2011/01/11/pkg.cohen.baby. jenny.update.cnn#/video/health/2011/01/11/pkg.cohen.baby.jenny.update. cnn.

[4]Cappon, R. Fortune in sunburn cream. *The News and Courier*, July 11, 1949.

[5]Tucker, A. Tender mercies: Mary Catherine Bunting—former nun, nurse, and philanthropist—gives her time and money from the heart. *The Baltimore Sun*, December 26, 2007.

[6]Fowler, G. Harry Weinberg, 82, businessman in transit and real estate, is dead. *The New York Times*, November 6, 1990.

[7]Olesker, M. Weinberg's life gave few clues to final kind act. *The Baltimore Sun*, November 6, 1990.

[8]Ibid.

[9]Ibid.

[10]Roylance, F. D. Rich recluse assured his privacy in death. *The Baltimore Evening Sun*, November 6, 1990.

[11]Surgery often has unexpected benefits. See Trivedi, B. P. The Bypass Cure. *Discover,* December 2012.

[12]Woods, M. New surgery helps liver cancer patients. *Toledo Blade*, June 13, 1989. Minton's other accomplishments include developing the laser as a surgical tool and using CGA antigen levels to detect malignancies.

Four

[1]Pollack, A. Hot chemotherapy bath: patients see hope, critics hold doubts. *The New York Times*, August 12, 2011, updated October 12, 2011. This article is sometimes archived under a newer headline, "Heated, Harrowing Chemotherapy Bath May Be Only Hope for Some."

[2]According to Jennifer Francis, Mercy practice manager, all insurance companies have a standard of care, which can be found online. That standard, however, generally isn't updated until a case forces the issue. If an insurance company that never had approved a HIPEC surgery is asked to do so, medical personnel at the company supposedly will survey the current literature and come to a decision.

[3]Ryan, D. P. Cytoreductive surgery and hyperthermic intraperitonal chemotherapy: history repeating itself or a new standard? *American Society of Clin-*

ical Oncology 1092–9118/10/1–10. For Sugarbaker's side of the debate, see Sugarbaker, P. H. Achieving long-term survival with cytoreductive surgery and perioperative chemotherapy to peritoneal surfaces for metastatic colon cancer. *American Society of Clinical Oncology* 1092–9118/10/1–10. See also Bath, C. Hot chemotherapy generates heated debate about its use with cytoreductive surgery to manage peritoneal metastasis. *ASCO Post*, October 15, 2011. As per ASCO's guidelines, Dr. Ryan declared a conflict of interest in the case, as he had given expert testimony in a related malpractice suit. Taking his side of the debate could only further Ryan's status as an expert in this respect.

[4]Berry, D. A. et al. High-dose chemotherapy with autologous stem-cell support as adjuvant therapy in breast cancer: overview of 15 randomized trials. *Journal of Clinical Oncology* 29(24):3214–23.

[5]Mukherjee, S. 2010, 321–328. The articles that stirred such high hopes include: Ariad, S. and W. R. Bezwoda. High-dose chemotherapy: therapeutic potential in the age of growth factor support. *Israel Journal of Medical Sciences* 28(6):377–85; Bezwoda, W. R., L. Seymour, and R. D. Dansey. High-dose chemotherapy with hematopoietic rescue as primary treatment for metastatic breast cancer: a randomized trial. *Journal of Clinical Oncology* 13(10): 2483–89; Bezwoda, W.R. High-dose chemotherapy with hematopoietic rescue in breast cancer. *Hematology and Cell Therapy* 41(2): 58–65; and the denouement, Weiss, R. B. et al. High-dose chemotherapy for high-risk primary breast cancer: an on-site review of the Bezwoda study. *The Lancet* 355(9208):999–1003.

[6]Ryan, D. P. Cytoreductive surgery and hyperthermic intraperitonal chemotherapy: history repeating itself or a new standard? *American Society of Clinical Oncology* 1092–9118/10/1–10.

[7]Radioactive iodine is also referred to as radioiodine remnant ablation, or I-131, or even I^{131}. The radioactive iodine not only can kill cancerous cells in the immediate area of the surgery but also those that have migrated to the lymph nodes or other parts of the body.

[8]Einhorn, L. E. Treatment of testicular cancer: a new and improved model. *American Society of Clinical Oncology* 8:1771–1781. In 1844 the remarkable Michele Peyrone, who was an Italian born to a wealthy family—and who went from being a physician treating patients in the European cholera epidemic of 1835, to being a chemist, to being an agricultural scientist who did important work in the development of fertilizers, in an attempt to synthesize a known compound, Magnus' green salt—also synthesized a yellow compound with completely different properties, cisplatin. When Peyrone passed away

in the 1880s, an article memorializing him noted that he felt it the duty of the rich to help the poor. See Fino, V. 1884. *Commemorazione del Prof. Michele Peyrone* in *Annali della Reale Accademia d'Agricoltura di Torino*, 23, 27. Also see the brief biography by George B. Kauffman et al. Michele Peyrone (1813–1883), discoverer of platinum. *Platinum Metals Review* 54(4): 250–256. In testicular cancer treatment, the initial combination of three agents was partly conceived to minimize the adverse side effects of each. Cisplatin caused nausea and kidney toxicity; vinblastine, bone-marrow toxicity; and bleomycin, lung toxicity. In the 1980s vinblastine was replaced by etoposide. It is still a bit of a mystery why cisplatin works so well on testicular cancer but hardly at all on any other cancer. Cisplatin was approved by the US Food and Drug Administration in 1978.

[9]Malone D. L. et al. Blood transfusion, independent of shock severity, is associated with worse outcome in trauma. Department of Surgery, University of Maryland School of Medicine and R. Adams Cowley Shock Trauma Center, Baltimore. *Journal of Trauma* 54(5):898–905, discussion 905–7. (2003).

[10]Dellinger R. P. et al. Surviving sepsis campaign guidelines for management of severe sepsis and septic shock. *Critical Care Medicine* 32(3):858–73. (2004). There is a caveat here, as one of the protocols may need to be revisited; see Maitland, K. et al. Mortality after fluid bolus in African children with severe infection. *The New England Journal of Medicine*, 364:2483–2495. (2011).

[11]Glasziou, P. et al. When are randomised trials unnecessary? Picking signal from noise. *British Medical Journal* 334(7589):339. (2007). Contributing also are Abdelhamid Attia, Benjamin Djulbegovic, Hywel Williams, Jan Vandenbrouke, Olad Dekkers, Dave Sackett, Jonathan Meakins, Ruth Gilbert, Amanda Burls, and Ken Fleming.

[12]Sugarbaker, P. H., as told to T. Bond. The evolution of treatment for peritoneal metastases. *Colorectal Cancer* 2(3):192. (2013).

[13]The undercover unit to study these gasses was called the Chemical Warfare Unit and was housed within the wartime Office of Scientific Research and Development. See Mukherjee S., 2010, 90. The Geneva Protocol of 1925 outlawed the use of mustard gas but not the stockpiling of it. In any event although the United States signed the protocol, they did not ratify it until the 1970s.

[14]Davis, D. 2007, 200. See also Krumbhaar, E. B. The role of the blood and the bone marrow in certain forms of gas poisoning. *Journal of the American Medical Association* lxxii:39. (1919). See also Pappenheimer, A. W. The ef-

fect of intravenous injection of dichlorethylsulphide on rabbits. *Proceedings of the Society for Experimental Biology and Medicine* xvi:92. (1919).

[15]DeVita Jr., V. T. and E. Chu. 2008. A history of cancer chemotherapy. *The Journal of Cancer Research.* 68:8643 (2008).

[16]Ibid.

[17]Davis, D. 2007, 203. See also, L. S. et al. Nitrogen mustard therapy. *Journal of the American Medical Association* 132:126–132. (1946).

[18] "Clinical, hematologic, and histologic details of 5 patients with acute leukemia treated with aminopterin, selected from a group of 16 patients so treated, form the basis of this paper. It is again emphasized that these remissions are temporary in character and that the substance is toxic and may be productive of even greater disturbances than have been encountered so far in our studies. No evidence has been mentioned in this report that would justify the suggestion of the term 'cure' of acute leukemia in children. A promising direction for further research concerning the nature and treatment of acute leukemia in children appears to have been established by the observations reported." Farber, S. et al. Temporary remissions in acute leukemia in children produced by folic acid antagonist, 4-aminopteroyl-glutamic acid (aminopterin). *New England Journal of Medicine* 238:787–793. Much more detail on Farber and his work can also be found in Siddhartha Mukherjee's Pulitzer Prize–winning *The Emperor of All Maladies: A Biography of Cancer.*

[19]Mukherjee, S. 2010, 219.

[20]One example should suffice to illustrate the enormity of the endeavor; on a trip to the Pacific Northwest in August 1962, a Cancer Chemotherapy National Service Center (CCNSC) botanist collected the bark from the Pacific yew tree, *Taxus brevifolia*, among many other samples. In tests in 1964, the bark was found to be poisonous. In September 1966, CCNSC chemists Monroe E. Wall and Mansukh C. Wani isolated the active ingredient in fresh samples of the yew bark, calling it "taxol." They announced their findings in June 1967 and published their results in 1971. In 1977 the decision was made to do experiments with taxol on leukemic mice, but there were two problems—it took a lot of bark to produce a small amount of taxol, and no one had yet been able to synthesize the compound. Nonetheless the CCNSC ordered seven thousand pounds of yew bark. In 1978 taxol was demonstrated to be mildly effective in the mice, and in 1979 pharmacologist Susan B. Horwitz created further interest with her publication. (See Schiff, P. B., J. Fant, and S. B. Horwitz. Promotion of microtubule assembly *in vitro* by taxol. *Nature* 277:665–667, doi:10.1038/277665a0). This paper showed taxol had a

previously unknown mechanism involving the stabilization of microtubules. The animal studies were completed in June 1982, and the agency prepared for clinical trials on humans. Phase I clinical trials began in 1984, with the Phase II trials planned in 1985. They did not start until the end of 1986, however, as more bark was needed; they commissioned the collection of twelve thousand more pounds. After May 1988 reports that showed taxol had some effectiveness in both melanoma patients and those with ovarian cancer, one National Cancer Institute specialist, Gordon Cragg, estimated they might need to harvest as many as 360,000 trees annually. This ultimately had two results: 1) the NCI sought a partner and selected Bristol-Myers Squibb; and 2) taxol was successfully synthesized. In 1990 Bristol-Myers Squib applied to trademark taxol with a new generic name of paclitaxel. The trademark was approved in 1992, as was the company's new drug application. Bristol-Myers Squib had exclusive marketing rights for five years, with sales eventually reaching $1.6 billion by 2000. The entire story, complete with legal complications, can be further explored in Jordan Goodman and Vivien Walsh's 2001 book *The Story of Taxol: Nature and Politics in the Pursuit of an Anti-Cancer Drug.*

[21]Nausea is a curious thing, but it also can be a many splendored thing. In Steve Martin's movie *Roxanne* (1987), inspired by Edmond Rostand's play *Cyrano de Bergerac* (1897), the character of Chris McDonnell becomes nauseous at the sight of a beautiful woman, a rare but real phenomena. In fact any number of things can make a person feel nauseous, including seasickness, motion sickness, certain odors, the sight of blood, and the thought of getting an injection; even the thought of getting nauseous itself can cause nausea, which has been given the clinical name of "anticipatory nausea," with as many as 29 percent of chemo patients experiencing it.

The true curiosity is not that nausea has so many causes but that intuitively it seems to arise from the gut; in fact it arises from the brain—specifically from the chemoreceptor trigger zone (CTZ), which lies at the center of the brain. The stimulus for nausea may indeed come from the stomach, or it may come from the inner ear, feelings, sensations, or chemicals or radiation. Except for antacids that are sometimes taken in addition to other drugs, most anti-nausea drugs in use today target the brain. Also, every chemotherapy drug has been rated as to its *emetic* potential, or how nauseous it will make a patient feel. (See McKay, J. and T. Schacher. 2009. *The Chemotherapy Survival Guide,* third edition, Oakland, CA: New Harbinger Publications, 69–70, 77.)

[22]See DeVita Jr., V. T. and E. Chu. 2008. Also see Mukherjee, S. 2010, 135–138, 168, 219.

Five

[1]Brady, M. My doctor saved my life! *Angie's List*, March 2012.

[2]See Coley W. B. *Annals of Surgery 1891* 14:199–200 (1887) and Gresser, I. A. Chekhov, M.D., and Coley's toxins. *New England Journal of Medicine* 317(7):457, PMID 3302707.

[3]See also Coley W. B. The Treatment of malignant tumors by repeated innoculations of erysipelas: with a report of ten original cases. *American Journal of the Medical Sciences* 10:487–511 (1893) and Hobohm, U. Fever therapy revisited. *British Journal of Cancer* 92:421–425. (2005).

[4]It's possible that some of the skepticism in Coley's time was a matter of economics. His patient, Elizabeth Dashiell, was the younger sister of a childhood friend of John D. Rockefeller, Jr., the only son of the founder of Standard Oil. Rockefeller contributed generously to Coley's research after her death, and the Memorial Hospital attached to the Sloan-Kettering Institute in Manhattan is a direct result of his philanthropy. (See Stephen S. Hall, *A Commotion in the Blood*, 1997).

[5]Hart, G. D. Descriptions of blood and blood disorders before the advent of laboratory studies. *British Journal of Haematology* 115(4):719-28. (2001).

[6]Mukherjee, S. 2010, 466.

[7]The Goldie-Coleman hypothesis calls for non-crossresistant drugs to be used in lower doses in combination. Competing is the Norton-Simon hypothesis, which calls for maximum tolerated doses delivered in sequence.

[8]Ziegler, J. L., I. T. Magrath, and C. L. Olweny. Cure of Burkitt's lymphoma: ten-year follow-up of 157 Ugandan patients. *The Lancet* 2(8149):936–8. (1979). See also Ziegler, J. L. et al. Combined modality treatment of Burkitt's lymphoma. *Cancer Treatment Report* 62(12):2031–4. (1978).

See also Friedman H. S. Rational[e] for "eight-in-one" chemotherapy. *Journal of Clinical Oncology* 6(2)393–395. (1988).

Glossary

abdominopelvic cavity The abdominal and pelvic cavities combined.

adjuvant therapy When treatment, usually chemotherapy, is used *after* all visible tumor has been removed through surgery. From the Latin for "toward" and "help." Coined by Paul Carbone at the NIH in the mid-1960s. Contrast to neoadjuvant therapy, which can be radiation or chemotherapy administered prior to surgery.

anesthetics Drugs used to relieve pain, make a part of the body numb (local anesthetics), or cause unconsciousness (general anesthetics). Today's anesthetics are primarily based on the nineteenth-century work of Joseph Lister.

antibiotics Any of a large group of chemical substances produced by microorganisms and fungi that can be used to fight infection and disease. Those substances that fight infection and disease that are synthetic or semisynthetic are instead called "antibacterials." The term *antibiotics* was coined by biochemist and microbiologist Selman Waksman in 1942.

antibody

A protein made by white blood cells in fighting infection and disease. Antibodies also can be introduced to the body through infusion, injection, or oral medication.

antigen

A substance that produces one or more antibodies. Short for "antibody generator."

apoptosis

The termination of a cell, a process that is unvaried. Cellular membranes are disrupted; the cytoplasmic and nuclear skeletons are broken down; the cytosol is extruded; the chromosomes are degraded; and the nucleus is fragmented. This takes a half hour to two hours. Last the cell corpse is engulfed by nearby cells and disappears, usually within twenty four hours. (See Wylie, A. H., J. F. Kerr, and A. R. Currie, Cell death: the significance of apoptosis. *International Review of Cytology*, 68:251-306.)

appendiceal cancer   See PMP.

appendix cancer   See PMP.

argon beam coagulator   A pen-like instrument that sprays argon gas on surgically cut tissue, creating quick coagulation and reducing blood loss.

ascites   An accumulation of extra fluid in the abdominal cavity. Fluid in the cavity acts as a lubricant and is normally secreted then absorbed, but a breakdown in either activity can lead to ascites.

B cells   One of the lymphocytes, the others being T cells and natural killer (NK) cells. The B refers to the bursa in birds, whose bones are hollow, and the bone marrow in mammals, even though all blood cells are made in the bone marrow. B cells circulate in both the blood system and the lymphatic system, performing the function of immune surveillance. They need a signal from the T cells to be activated.

basophil

Only about one in ten thousand white blood cells is a basophil, and it serves several functions, including ensuring that blood does not clot too quickly.

benign

Not malignant or cancerous. Some tumors, usually lumps felt beneath the skin, are benign, but all cancer is malignant. From the Latin for "well" and "produce" as well as Middle English and Old French for "good by nature."

beta blockers

A class of drugs prescribed for hypertension and sometimes after the occurrence of a heart attack. They work primarily by blocking adrenaline and noradrenaline.

biopsy

When tissue from a tumor is extracted from the body. This can be done with a needle or through minor surgery.

blind(ed) study

When a clinical study is randomized, with an equal number of patients receiving two (occasionally more than two) treatments. When the study is blinded, the patient does not know which treatment is being used. When possible, the doctor will not know the treatment as well, created a double-blinded study. Blinded studies are an effort to eliminate bias from the results.

blood count

A count of the white blood cells (which generally fight infection and disease), red blood cells (which carry nutrients and oxygen), and platelets (which cause clotting). This is a valuable tool to track a patient's progress and determine whether he or she is ready to withstand a procedure (surgery or chemotherapy, for example). Counts are expressed as a number per cubic millimeter. The following counts are generally considered normal: white, 4,300 to 10,800, with an average of about 5,000; red, about 5.4 million for an adult male, a bit less for females; platelets, 150,000–400,000.

blood transfusion

In surgery blood loss is often compensated for with a blood transfusion (blood donated by another individual). White blood cells are always removed from transfused blood, and a protocol for matching blood types is used. There are A, B, AB, and O blood types, with O blood being universally accepted by the immune system. In addition each of these blood types can be Rh+ or Rh-, making a total of eight blood types. Today, blood transfusions are safer than ever, with the odds of acquiring HIV about 1 in 1.5 million.

bone marrow

Located within the bones, this produces all blood cells. Author and oncologist Siddhartha Mukerjee refers to it as an organ, in truth.

bone-marrow transplant

This procedure is recommended if a patient's bone marrow is not producing new blood cells, and for cancers it is generally confined to leukemia (cancer of the white blood cells), lymphoma, and instances in which chemotherapy has destroyed the bone marrow. In some instances the patient's own bone marrow is frozen prior to chemotherapy; in others, a donor who is a good genetic match is needed. Stem cells also can be used.

cancer

(Also known as "carcinoma" or "neoplasm.") A disease of uncontrolled cell growth that disturbs nearby tissue and can invade other parts of the body through the bloodstream or lymphatic system. Individual cancers, such as lung cancer, pancreatic cancer, etc., are named after their place of origin. Cancer cells are distinguished from normal cells in six ways: 1) cancer cells grow without a signal from the body; 2) they

do not respond to antigrowth
instructions; 3) they can spread
through the body; 4) there are no
limits to their ability to replicate
themselves; 5) they can recruit
other cells to create a blood
supply; 6) they evade natural
death. (See Hanahan, D. and
R. A. Weinberg. The hallmarks
of cancer. *Cell* 100:57–70.)
"Cancer," penned by the
encyclopedist Aulus Cornelius
Celsus, comes from the Roman
for "crab."

cancer staging

For a doctor to recommend
treatment, cancer is first given
a numeric rating of one (I)
to four (IV), with IV being
the most advanced state.
The staging is done through
physical exams, scans, and
blood tests. In pathological
staging, tissue is removed in a
biopsy for examination by a
pathologist.

carcinoma

Cancer that starts in the skin
or the tissue that lines internal
organs. Penned by the Greek

242

physician Hippocrates, the word is derived from the Greek for "crab."

carcinomatosis

The state of multiple carcinomas in the same site or system, originating along the epithelial surfaces then spreading. Peritoneal carcinomatosis of the abdominopelvic cavity is one type, but there are others.

carcinosis

See carcinomatosis.

cardiologist

A heart specialist, derived from the Greek for "heart."

CAT scan

The original name of today's CT scan. Short for "computer axial tomography."

CBC

Short for "complete blood count test." This test measures the number of red and white blood cells, the amount of hemoglobin (a protein that carries oxygen and contains iron), and usually the platelet count. The results can reflect a patient's problems with fluid volume (such as dehydration). The test also can reveal problems with red blood cell production or help diagnose infections, allergies, and problems with blood clotting.

chemotherapy
The use of toxic chemicals to kill cancer cells, as opposed to the use of radiation, or as opposed to more recent strategies, such as hormone therapy or targeted therapy. Chemotherapy developed after the effects of mustard gas were reviewed, and today we have multiple agents with an almost infinite number of possible combinations. The term was coined in 1907 by German biochemist and Nobel Prize winner Paul Ehrlich.

chromosome
A thread-like body that carries genetic information. Humans have twenty-three pairs of chromosomes. The literal meaning from the Greek is "colored body," and the term was coined in the 1880s.

cirrhosis

Diseases that kill liver cells can lead to cirrhosis, an abnormal structure and function of the liver. Though the disease is often associated with alcohol use, there are many causes, including fat, certain medications, viruses, genetically linked diseases, and even attacks from the immune system itself. Cirrhosis can be a serious condition, as it can prevent the liver from cleansing the blood supply, providing clotting agents, and performing other functions. The word has been in use since the 1830s and comes from the Greek for "orange-tawny."

cisplatin

One of more than fifty chemotherapeutic agents. First synthesized in 1844, it was approved by the FDA for cancer treatment in 1978. It is a bit of a puzzle why this drug has had spectacular results on testicular cancer but has had little effect on other cancers.

clinical benefit

The benefit received by patients in clinical trials. Coined in the 1990s by Doctor Gordon Guyatt.

clinical study

A clinical study includes all clinical trials but also can include surveys that don't include testing for a variable. Some studies are retroactive; for example, in the determination of which candidates are likely to be successfully treated, all the known factors of previous patients may be examined.

clinical trial

The testing of a new drug, a new purpose for an existing drug, a new dosage, a new technique, a new procedure, or even a new treatment altogether. Usually the change being considered in a trial is compared to the old standard. Sometimes clinical trials are referred to as "clinical studies"; this is not inaccurate, but there are many studies that are not considered trials. Clinical trials that are currently open can be accessed on the NIH webpage.

CMP   Comprehensive metabolic
                           panel blood test. This measures
                           kidney and liver function,
                           glucose (sugar) and protein
                           levels, electrolytes, and acid/
                           base balance in the blood. It is
                           a diagnostic tool that includes
                           fourteen standardized tests and is
                           routinely ordered up for annual
                           physicals.

colonoscope   A flexible, lighted, tubular
                           instrument that uses fiber optics
                           to permit visualization of the
                           colon.

colostomy   A procedure that reroutes the
                           colon through a surgically
                           produced opening in the
                           abdominal wall, usually because
                           of the removal of a diseased
                           portion of the lower intestine.
                           This is different from an
                           ileostomy, in which the entire
                           colon is removed.

colorectal cancer   Cancer of the lining of the colon
                           or rectum.

complete blood count test   See CBC.

comprehensive metabolic panel blood test   See CMP.

Conn's disease   (Also called "primary aldosteronism" or "PA.") Conn's disease occurs when one or both adrenal glands produce too much of the hormone aldosterone, which in turn creates a buildup of sodium, accompanied by high blood pressure and a loss of potassium. Measuring renin and aldosterone levels, followed by adrenal vein sampling, in which blood is drawn from both adrenal veins, can help pinpoint the problem.

CT scan   Short for computed tomography. During this procedure a computer reassembles multiple X-ray images to develop a two-dimensional image. For example an X-ray couldn't capture a horizontal plane in the abdomen, but a CT scan could.

cytoreductive surgery   The removal of all or almost all of the visible tumors in the abdominopelvic cavity. The techniques Doctor Armando Sardi uses to accomplish this are use of a laser, use of electro-evaporation, use of ultrasonic dissection, and use of an argon beam coagulator. The surgery lasts ten to fourteen hours or longer. The surgery can involve the complete or partial removal of organs, including segments of the large and small bowel, the spleen, the stomach, and the liver. The surgery also can involve a complete hysterectomy. Because very small tumors (less than two millimeters in complete cytoreductive surgery, scored CØ, C1, C2, C3, or C4) and microscopic cancer cells can be left behind, HIPEC is often administered immediately after surgery, though some centers do not heat the chemotherapeutic solution.

cytotoxic Poisonous to plant or animal cells.

Data Safety Monitoring Board See DSMB.

debulking surgery

In situations where all of the tumor cannot be removed, surgeons remove as much tumor as possible, with the idea that subsequent systemic chemotherapy would then be more effective. The term is often used interchangeably with "cytoreductive surgery." It's not the same procedure, but it's possible that an attempt at cytoreductive surgery could end up as an exercise in debulking.

dendritic cells

A white blood cell that processes antigens and acts as a messenger between the innate and adaptive immunity systems.

deep venous thrombosis

See DVT.

diagnosis

The process of identifying a disease. Cancer is definitively identified by a pathologist who examines tissue taken during a biopsy. The medical usage of the word dates from the 1680s and comes from the Greek for "apart" and "to learn."

diagnostician

A doctor who makes a diagnosis, or a doctor who specializes in making diagnoses.

dianeal solution

Chemotherapeutic agents are mixed into this solution during HIPEC.

distillate

A concentrated essence.

diuretic

Any substance that promotes the production of urine.

DNA

Short for "deoxyribonucleic acid." The material that carries our genetic code and is found in nearly all cells in the human body.

DNA profiling

(Also called "gene typing," "DNA testing," and "genetic fingerprinting.") This is a technique best known for identifying paternity and is a medical option available to patients because specific gene markers are associated with certain diseases, such as breast cancer. Profiles generate probabilities, not certainty, but

DNA profiling is nonetheless considered a useful tool. Genetic profiling was pioneered by Sir Alec Jeffreys and first reported in 1984. The cost of profiling has dropped dramatically in the last decade and is sometimes covered by insurance.

DNA testing   See DNA profiling.

DSMB   Data Safety Monitoring Board. In large clinical trials, this is an independent board that helps ensure the integrity of the data and provides an additional layer of safety for the patients. If one of two treatments proves clearly inferior, or clearly superior, before the clinic trial is completed, the DSMB is responsible for ending the trial early.

DVT   Deep venous thrombosis. A blood clot that forms in a deep vein, usually in the calves or thighs. There are any number of causes or factors, including prolonged surgery. Preventative measures

are now the standard in surgeries
that last forty-five minutes
or more, and tightly wrapped
Ace bandages or compression
stockings and leg exercises are
recommended after surgery.

DVT compression therapy A broad range of practices, from
the use of specialized equipment
during surgery, to the use of Ace
bandages and stockings, to the
prescription of certain medicines,
such as anticoagulants.

ECG See EKG.

effectiveness (in medicine) How well a
treatment works in the everyday
practice of medicine. Compare to
"efficacy" below.

efficacy How well a treatment works
in clinical studies or other
laboratory settings.

EKG Electrocardiography. A
noninvasive procedure that
measures the electrical activity
of the heart and can give an
indication regarding how

healthy the heart is. Generally ten electrodes are placed on the body, one on each ankle, one on each wrist, and six on the torso. The word "electrocardiography" was coined in the early twentieth century from the Greek for "electric," "heart," and "to write."

electrocardiography   See EKG.

embolism   A potentially fatal blood clot, often as a result of inactivity. The most common embolisms are pulmonary embolisms and those that form in the legs. The word was first used in England in 1855 and comes from the Greek for "stopper."

endocrine system   A series of glands that secrete hormones into the bloodstream and regulate many functions, including metabolism, growth, tissue function, and mood. The term was coined in the early twentieth century and comes from the Greek for "inside" and "secrete."

endocrinologist   An endocrine-system specialist.

endoscope   An instrument used to look inside the body without making an incision. The light source is typically outside the body and is delivered via filter optics. The parts of the endoscope consist of the lens system, the eyepiece, a rigid or flexible tube, sometimes a means of suction, and an additional channel to allow entry of medical instruments. The endoscope can be used to examine the stomach, intestines, urinary tract, and uterus, among other hollow organs. The word was coined in the 1860s.

endoscopic mucosal resection   A technique, using an endoscope, to remove cancer from the gastrointestinal tract without creating an incision or damaging the organ. Considered minimally invasive.

endoscopic submucosal resection   A technique, using an endoscope, to remove cancer without creating an incision or damaging the organ. Considered minimally invasive. Often required for larger lesions.

endoscopy

An examination of the inner body with an endoscope and without the use of an incision.

enterostomal therapy

Care for the stoma and education regarding an appropriate diet.

eosinophil

A white blood cell that combats multicellular parasites and certain infections.

epidemiologist

A practitioner of epidemiology

epidemiology

The science concerned with the study of the factors that determine and influence the frequency and distribution of disease, injury, and other health-related events and their causes in a defined human population. From the Greek for "among" and "the people."

epithelial cells

These cells line the surfaces of tissues and organs throughout the body.

erysipelas infection   An infection that can cause fever, chills, headache, nausea, and skin lesions that can resemble an orange peel. There have been several observations that this infection can cause the remission of cancer. The modern name for this infection is Streptococcus pyogenes.

esophagoscope   A flexible instrument inserted through the mouth to create a visualization of the esophagus.

estrogen   A female hormone. Along with the male hormone testosterone, it is used as hormone therapy for the treatment of a few cancers.

evidence-based medicine   Medical practice based on the results of clinical trials. In the loosest sense, evidence-based medicine has been with us a long time, but it has only become the standard, as opposed to tradition-based therapy, since the 1970s. Beer and Axmaker give much credit to the Scottish epidemiologist Archie Cochrane in the writing of *Effectiveness &*

Efficiency: Random Reflections on Health Services, published in 1972. (See T.M. Beer and L.W. Axmaker's 2012 book *Cancer Clinical Trials*, 15.)

experimental drug

(Also known as an "investigational drug.") A drug being tested in trials that has not yet been approved for other use by the FDA.

experimental medicine

Whereas the term "experimental drug" has a specific meaning, "experimental medicine" does not. Herbal treatments, for example, can be called experimental, even if they've been used for thousands of years. The NIH lists standard therapies when they have been established.

FDA

Food and Drug Administration. A branch of the United States Department of Health and Human Services that oversees many activities and enforces laws to protect public health, most notably Section 361 of the Public

Health Service Act of 1944.
Today's FDA was created in
1906 by the Wiley Act and was
originally called the Food, Drug,
and Insecticide Administration.
The FDA's 2013 budget request
was for approximately $4.5
billion.

fibrin
A white, insoluble, elastic protein
formed when blood clots.

fistula
An abnormal opening between
one hollow organ and another,
or between a hollow organ and
the surface of the skin, generally
caused by disease. From the
Latin for "pipe" or "tube."

FOLFOX
A specific chemotherapeutic
mix that consists of neoadjuvant
5- fluorouracil, folinic acid, and
oxaliplatin. The rationale in
using FOLFOX is to combine
the effectiveness of the agents
while at the same time diluting
the harmful side effects of
each. FOLFOX is administered
intravenously. (You may see
individual protocols for delivery,

such as FOLFOX4, FOLFOX5, FOLFOX6, etc.)

Food and Drug Administration   See FDA.

fractional kill hypothesis   (Also known as "logkill hypothesis," "the Skipper-Schabel model," and even "the Skipper-Schabel-Wilcox model.") This hypothesis states that with each chemotherapy session, a fraction of the cancer cells are killed. In general if a chemotherapeutic solution can kill 99 percent of existing cells, six sessions would be needed to eliminate the cancer.

gastroenterology   The field of medicine relating to the digestive system and its disorders. From the Greek for "stomach," "intestine," and "reason."

gene therapy   A cancer treatment that uses DNA to treat disease. The most common form of gene therapy involves using DNA that encodes a functional gene in order to replace a mutated gene. Another strategy in gene therapy is to use healthy genes to "turn off" the runaway growth signals in cancerous genes. Gene therapy was cautiously proposed in 1972, making the field largely experimental. See Friedmann, T. and R. Roblin. Gene therapy for human genetic disease?" *Science* 175(4025):949.

gene typing   See DNA profiling.

genetic fingerprinting   See DNA profiling.

glycoprotein   A protein with a carbohydrate component that plays a role in cell-cell interactions.

gold standard   For a diagnostic test, the gold standard would be 100 percent accuracy, as measured by sensitivity and specificity. To be entirely sensitive, all patients who have a condition test positive for that condition. To be entirely specific, all patients who do not have a condition test negatively for the condition. Many diagnostic tests produce false positives or false negatives.

gynecology

The field covering the female reproductive system and its disorders. Coined in 1847 from the Greek for "study" and "women."

hematological

Of the blood. From the Greek for "blood."

HIPEC

(Also known as "hyperthermic intraperitoneal chemotherapy.") Used in conjunction with cytoreductive surgery, this is a heated chemotherapeutic solution (hot chemo bath) administered at 40–43° C (about 108° F), depending on the treatment center, with the patient temperature maintained at 37–38° C to prevent hyperthermia. The bath can last 30 to 120 minutes, again depending on the treatment center. In theory, the procedure should work for multiple reasons. The trauma of surgery produces fibrin, and cancer cells could embed themselves in the fibrin, escaping later intravenous chemotherapy. The chemo bath, applied directly to the surgical area, can attack cancer on the surface of the organs, as well as on the surface of the peritoneum, a thin membrane that encases the abdominopelvic cavity, with trace amounts also absorbed into the bloodstream. Also the blood supply for cancer cells is not as robust as it is for normal cells, so heat alone, at the right temperature, can kill cancer cells without harming normal cells. As with almost all therapies that involve chemotherapeutic solutions, results are not uniform.

histology

The examination of tissue through a microscope or electron microscope, with the tissue often made more visible by staining. In medicine the technique is used to confirm cancer and identify specific cancers. From the Greek for "tissue" and "logic."

hormonal therapy

A therapy that targets hormones to act as a catalyst. Hormone blockers, synthetic hormones, or other agents are used to interfere with natural hormones to slow cancer growth in certain cases, such as breast cancer or prostate cancer.

hormones

Chemicals that circulate in the blood and cause specific reactions. In males, for example, testosterone is associated with the development of the testis and prostate gland and also promotes muscle mass, bone mass, and hair. In females, estrogen, which has three variants that affect the stages of the female life cycle, regulates the reproductive cycle and breast development. There are many hormones besides testosterone and estrogen, and they can affect such things as hunger, sexual desire, mood, growth, activation or inhibition of the immune system, the fight-or-flight mechanism, and the preparation of the body for the puberty, pregnancy, and menopause. From the Greek for "impetus."

hospice care

A form of palliative care given to patients who could succumb to death within six months and are no longer receiving treatment for their cancer. The goal is to help patients live as well and as long as possible. Doctors must sign off on this in order for insurance to cover it. Hospice care can continue indefinitely, and some patients "graduate" from hospice care, either because their condition improves or because new treatment becomes available.

hyperplasia

An increase in the number of cells or a proliferation of cells. Hyperplasia can cause tumors and is only sometimes an indication of disease. This condition can occur naturally, such as when an expectant mother is getting ready to nurse. Coined in the 1860s, it comes from the Greek words meaning "over" and "formation."

Compare to "hypertrophy," when cell size increases, and "neoplasia" or cancer.

hyperthermia

An elevated body temperature that demands immediate medical attention. The most common causes are heat stroke and an adverse drug reaction, but there are others. Coined in the 1880s. Compare to "fever," which may or may not be a medical emergency.

hyperthermic intraperitoneal chemotherapy

See HIPEC.

hypertrophy

A condition in which cell size increases. Hypertrophy can occur naturally, as with bodybuilding, or artificially, as when an individual takes steroids. Coined between 1825 and 1835.

hysterectomy

The removal of the uterus from the female body. A complete hysterectomy includes the removal of the cervix as well. Coined in 1886 from the Greek meaning "womb" and "cutting out."

ileostomy

The creation of an artificial opening from the ileum through the abdominal wall in order to permit drainage of the contents of the small intestine.

immune system

The system in the human body that fights infection and maintains the body's good health. The first line of defense is the skin itself, which puts up a physical barrier. Important components consist of the lymphatic system and leukocytes, the latter an umbrella term used for various white blood cells. Humans have between five hundred and six hundred lymph nodes, with about half of them clustered in the neck and the other half clustered in the underarms, groin, chest, and abdomen. The clinical significance of the lymph nodes is that when they are inflamed it can mean anything from a throat infection to cancer. With cancer the lymph node status is so significant that it is used for cancer staging, which in turn helps determine both treatment and prognosis. Also these lymph nodes are packed with lymphocytes and macrophages, two different white blood cells. In addition to the skin, the immune system has two other lines of defense. One is called the autoimmune system and can more or less be thought of as innate. The second is the acquired-immunity system, which creates an immunological memory after an initial response to a specific pathogen; traditionally vaccines are created by effectively manipulating this memory. From the Latin for "exempt from public service."

immunotherapy   The treatment of disease by inducing, enhancing, or suppressing an immune response.

in situ   A cancer that has not metastasized, also called a noninvasive cancer. From the Latin for "in place."

in vitro When experimentation takes place outside a living body, often in a test tube or a petri dish. To see whether a particular agent has an effect on a particular type of cancer cell, for example, the interaction can be studied in isolation. Compare to "in vivo." "In vitro" comes from Latin for "within the glass."

in vivo When experimentation takes place inside a living body, often murine models (rats and mice). The advantage here is that when an agent is tested on a particular cancer, for example, the effect of all of the body's systems also can be monitored, thus a more complete picture arises than from in vitro studies alone. In vivo studies on two different species are now compulsory before experiments can be performed on humans, a safety precaution. Compare to "in vitro." "In vivo" comes from the Latin for "within the living."

informed consent

A policy designed to protect the patient. Before any medical procedure or experiment can be performed on a patient, the patient must be informed of the benefits and drawbacks of the procedure, then must sign a legal document giving the doctor or center permission to proceed.

intraperitoneal chemotherapy

When a solution, heated or unheated, is administered directly into the abdominal cavity. Much higher doses can be administered this way than can be administered intravenously.

investigational drug

See experimental drug.

IV

(Short for "intravenous catheter.") A hollow needle that is fastened to the skin and enters the vein for the purpose of maintaining hydration, sometimes providing nutrients, sometimes providing medicine, etc. An IV also can be used to draw blood.

laparoscope   The key device used in laparoscopic surgery.

laparoscopic surgery   (Also called "minimally invasive surgery," "MIS," or "keyhole surgery.") A surgery in which small incisions are made to the abdomen; the area for surgery is illuminated by a cold light source (halogen or xenon); and the area is projected onto a screen. The procedure causes less pain for the patient, promotes a quicker recovery time, and has cosmetic advantages. Compare to "laparotomy," when a large incision is made. From the Greek for "flank."

laparotomy   (Also known as "celiotomy.") This exploratory surgery requires a large incision through the abdominal wall. The technique also can be used as a first step in a regular surgery. Compare to "laparoscopy," which requires a small incision. From the Greek for "flank."

leukemia Cancer of the white blood cells. Coined in 1855 by Rudolph Virchow, from the Greek for "white."

leukocytes White blood cells. Coined in 1870 from the Greek for "white."

lymph nodes Gland-like masses of tissue that are an integral part of the immune system.

lymphatic system A system of five hundred to six hundred lymph nodes in the body that are an integral part of the immune system.

lymphocyte A type of white blood cell.

magic bullet The ideal therapeutic agent, one that would kill all of a given pathogen but would spare all other cells. Originally coined by German physician Paul Ehrlich around the turn of the twentieth century, but its usage in English may date from the 1960s.

magnetic resonance imaging   See MRI.

malignant   When a tumor is malignant, it is characterized by uncontrolled growth and usually requires treatment. A malignant tumor is also called "invasive" or "metastatic," as its growth invades other sites in the body. Used in medicine since 1568, when it referred to the Bubonic Plague, it comes from the French for "malign," or "having an evil nature," and possibly the Latin "malignus," badly born.

maximum-tolerated dose   The highest dose that can be used that will produce a desired effect without unacceptable toxicity. Generally one of the goals of Phase I trials is to determine the maximum tolerated dose. Dosages begin low in testing and are increased incrementally until unacceptable toxicity is reached.

melphalan   A member of the nitrogen mustard class, this is one of over fifty chemotherapeutic agents.

mesothelioma

A malignant cancer that forms around the chest, abdomen, or heart, often associated with exposure to asbestos, a material used in building materials such as shingles, or floor tiles. HIPEC is used in treating peritoneal mesothelioma. Coined around the turn of the twentieth century.

metastasis

When disease-producing organisms or cancer migrate to other parts of the body through the bloodstream or lymphatic system. From the Greek for "transference," "removal," or "change" it also has been translated "beyond stillness."

mitomycin C

A chemotherapeutic agent that is particularly effective when administered topically after bladder resection; it has had other successes as well. Highly toxic, especially to bone marrow.

monocyte

A white blood cell that plays several roles. About half the body's monocytes are stored in the spleen.

MRI

A noninvasive medical imaging technology that uses radio waves and powerful magnetic fields to make the interior of the human body visible in three dimensions and in real time. Armenian-American physician Raymond Damadian built the first MRI machine in 1972.

mucin

Any of a group of glycoproteins that are found especially in the secretions of mucus membranes. It is similar to mucus.

mutation

A permanent change in genetic material that can sometimes be inherited by the next generation.

narcotic drugs

A medically imprecise term that refers to substances that initially bring exhilaration but ultimately produce inertia or apathy and insensibility. In medicine agents that are nonnarcotic are preferred so the patient does not become addicted to them. From the Greek for "I benumb."

nasogastric tube   See NG tube.

National Institutes   See NIH.
of Health

natural killer cells   See NK cells.

neoadjuvant therapy   Therapy, radiation, or chemotherapy administered to a patient prior to surgery. Compare to "adjuvant therapy."

neoplasm   (Also referred to as a "tumor.") An uncontrolled or abnormal growth of cells, often first recognized by swelling. Some tumors are benign, which means they are no longer growing and are considered harmless; some are malignant, still in the process of growing or spreading, and are considered dangerous. The word dates to the midnineteenth century, coined by Rudolph Virchow.

neuropathy   Loss of sensation, sometimes partial. In many cases sensation can be restored.

neutrophil

The most abundant of the white blood cells. In the event of inflammation, especially inflammation caused by bacterial infection, these are the first responders.

NG tube

A tube inserted through the nostril and that runs down to the stomach. It is used for draining the stomach of acids, generally during the period of time when the patient is receiving nutrients intravenously.

NIH

National Institutes of Health, an agency of the United States Department of Health and Human Services, centered in Bethesda, Maryland. The NIH has twenty-seven separate institutes, agencies, and offices and funds massive amounts of biomedical research, with a 2013 budget of about $29 billion after sequestration cuts. Though the NIH can trace its roots to the Marine Hospital Service formed in the 1790s, today's NIH was created by the Ransdell Act of 1930.

NK cells

Short for "natural killer cells." White blood cells that attack viruses around the third day of inflammation, inducing apoptosis (cell death). They serve to contain the virus until the adaptive immune system can generate a more long-lasting response.

obstetrics

The branch of medicine that revolves around childbirth and care for women giving childbirth.

ON-Q pump

The proprietary name of an appliance a patient can use to control pain. It is placed directly on the incision after surgery, is kept in place for about five days, and delivers a nonnarcotic numbing agent.

oncogene

A gene that has the potential to cause cancer. Oncogenes were first identified in viruses but are present in all cells. Some of the genes in each cell, when abnormally activated, can cause cancer. The term was coined in 1969 by NCI scientists Robert Huebner and George Todaro.

oncologist

One who studies cancer, which can include diagnosis and treatment. From the Greek for "swollen."

oncology

The study of cancer, which can include diagnosis and treatment. From the Greek for "swollen."

palliative care

The management of symptoms and side effects of cancer and cancer treatments, sometimes confused with hospice care, a branch of palliative care that deals with end-of-life issues. Palliative care can be offered or considered at any point in the cancer treatment process, including the earliest stages, and can be given concurrently with therapeutic treatment. Palliative care can consist of the same procedures as cancer treatment itself, such as surgery to relieve pain. Palliative care also can include interaction with psychologists, therapists, clergy, and support groups. From the Latin *"palliare,"* meaning "to cloak."

pathogen   (Also known as a "germ.") A microorganism such as a virus, bacterium, or fungi that can cause disease.

pathologist   One who studies pathology, often by identifying tissue. Surgeons and doctors often consult with pathologists. From the Greek "pathos," meaning "suffering."

pathology   The study of the cause, origin, or nature of disease, including changes that can be expected to occur as a result of the disease. Surgeons and doctors often consult with trained pathologists, who count X-rays, CT scans, MRIs, and microscopic views of tissue among their tools. Pathologists note the size of the tumor and where it originated based on the similarity or difference of the cells from normal cells, as well as the status of the corresponding lymph nodes. Pathologists also note the rate of growth of a tumor and whether the tumor is invasive. They also may test for changes in the DNA or for the presence of hormone receptors. The field of pathology appears to have come into existence in the late sixteenth century. From the Greek "*pathos*," meaning "suffering."

patient-controlled analgesia pump

See PCA pump.

PCA pump

Short for "patient-controlled analgesia pump." In some cases this pump is set to deliver a steady stream of pain medication intravenously, with the patient able to push a button for extra doses as needed; in other cases it delivers a dose only at the patient's bequest. The newer systems have a built in safeguard against an accidental overdose. Some advantages include immediate relief for the patient, and in many cases, less medication is used overall than in strictly timed dosages, a desired result in the use of narcotic drugs. Developed by Philip H. Sechzer in the late 1960s and described in 1971.

PCI

Peritoneal cancer index. A tool for prognosis that measures both the distribution and extent of cancer in thirteen abdominal and pelvic regions. Using the objective score, doctors can make predictions about the chances of complete cytoreduction and long-term survival. The maximum PCI score is thirty-nine. Obviously the lower the PCI score, the better the patient's chances are for survival. Introduced by Paul Sugarbaker and his associates no later than 1996.

perioperative chemotherapy

Chemotherapy given around the time of surgery, sometimes before and after, sometimes only after. The primary consideration revolves around which types of

cancer can be treated and which
regimens are best.

peritoneal cancer index See PCI.

peritoneal carcinomatosis An umbrella term for cancers
that have spread within the
peritoneum, regardless of where
they originated. These cancers
are usually heterogenous in
nature, with more than one type
of cancer cell present, making
successful treatment challenging.
"Primary peritoneal cancer"
refers to cancer that is thought
to originate on the peritoneal
surface itself.

peritoneal cavity This cavity lies below the
diaphragm and includes many
organs. The cavity is surrounded
by a thin, translucent abdominal
membrane called the peritoneum.
Cancer can be found anywhere
in this space, including on the
membrane itself. Cytoreductive
surgery is intended to remove
all the visible tumor, if possible.
From the Greek for "stretched
round."

peritoneal mesothelioma   An extremely rare cancer, with only two hundred to five hundred cases diagnosed in the United States each year. HIPEC is the only known treatment, though not all patients with peritoneal mesothelioma are good candidates for treatment. The only known cause of any kind of mesothelioma is asbestos, a building material that is now banned in many countries.

peritonectomy   Up to six procedures used to eliminate all visible tumor from the peritoneal cavity. Pioneered by Doctor Paul Sugarbaker and his associates.

peritoneum   The smooth translucent membrane that lines the abdominal cavity.

personalized medicine   Medical care built on the principle that individuals respond differently and uniquely to treatments and that treatments should be selected for each person based on an understanding of the unique biology of the disease and the patient's body.

PET scan　Positron emission tomography. A nuclear-imaging technology that can produce three-dimensional images, as opposed to X-rays and CT scans, which form two-dimensional images. About 90 percent of PET scans ordered are to determine whether a cancer has spread. Many individuals have contributed to this technology, which can be traced back to the late 1950s.

pharmacokinetics　See PK.

PK　Short for "pharmacokinetics." The study of how the body metabolizes any given drug, hormone, nutrient, or toxin. The metrics used have become standardized, but many of the measures are complex. From the Greek for "drug" and "motion."

PMP　(Also called "pseudomyxoma peritonei," "appendix cancer," or "appendiceal cancer.") The spread of mucin in the abdomen that originates with the appendix. There are multiple forms, not all of them cancerous, but even noncancerous PMP can be life threatening. From the Greek meaning "a false benign tumor embedded in mucus."

positron emission tomography

See PET scan.

prognosis

The likely outcome, or a range of likely outcomes, for any given patient based on the diagnosis and compared to other patients with the same or similar diagnosis, often expressed in percentages.

prostate cancer

Cancer of the prostate gland, part of the male reproductive system. It primarily affects men older than sixty. In an effort to detect it at an early stage, men can be screened with a PSA (prostate-specific antigen) blood test.

psychotropic drugs   (Also referred to as
                           "psychoactive drugs.") In
                           medicine these are drugs that
                           cross the blood-brain barrier and
                           can affect perception, mood,
                           cognition, and behavior. Such
                           drugs can bring comfort or
                           pleasure to the patient, and for
                           the same reason, they easily can
                           be abused.

radiofrequency ablation   A procedure that attempts to
                                destroy a tumor by a clinician
                                putting a thin electrode into
                                the tumor center and running
                                a current through it in order
                                to heat it. There are multiple
                                medical uses for this technology.
                                Introduced in 1987.

radiologist   A practitioner of radiology. From
                    the Latin "radius," meaning
                    "beam" or "ray."

radiology   The practice of interpreting
                  X-rays, CTs, PETs, MRIs, bone
                  scans, and ultrasounds. Based on
                  a radiologist's recommendation,
                  a biopsy may be ordered for

examination by a pathologist. From the Latin "radius," meaning "beam" or "ray."

randomized trial

A clinical trial in which everyone who signs up is randomly assigned to one of two (occasionally more than two) "arms." The arms can be two different procedures, two different drugs, two different dosages, etc. In order to eliminate bias in the results, the patient does not know in which arm he or she is in, and, when possible, the administrating doctor will not know either. The primary ethical concern in such a trial is that the patient should be informed of results from earlier trials and that the patient should be comfortable with being in either arm.

resection

(in medicine) Surgical removal of all or part of an organ, tissue, or structure.

Röntgen rays

A term used in parts of Europe for X-rays.

sarcoma

A cancer that develops in the bones or connecting tissue. Sarcomas make up about 1 percent of adult cancers and 15 percent of child cancers. They are usually found in the limbs but can be found in the abdomen, head, or neck. From the Greek for "fleshly growth."

scanxiety

The tension that builds among those who have or have had cancer as they move toward their regular checkup scan, with "hyperscanxiety" building up during the time they await the results. It is an imprecise medical term, and its usage is very recent.

screenings

(in medicine) Tests performed to detect cancer at an early stage, such as a routine colonoscopy, a routine mammogram, etc.

sensitivity

(in medicine) See gold standard.

signet ring cells

Malignant cancer cells that resemble signet rings and are associated with stomach, gallbladder, colon, breast, prostate, and ovarian cancer. Containing a lot of mucin, these cells are associated with a poorer prognosis.

specificity

(in medicine) See gold standard.

standard treatment

The best medical practice or procedure or medicine currently available. Since it is not necessarily the best practice possible, the standard treatment is often updated based on new evidence.

statistical significance

In general this is enough of a difference to almost rule out sheer chance. There are two different variables used in describing data, a- and p-, and in spite of the nuances, both give odds that a conclusion could be wrong. Usually, when the odds of a conclusion being wrong are less than 5 percent, the conclusion is said to be statistically significant. Coined in 1885 by statistician Sir Ronald Fisher.

stoma
An artificial opening in the body created by surgical means. Stomata (plural) can be made for the esophagus, urinary bladder, or gastrointestinal tract. The mouth is a natural stoma. From the Latin for "mouth."

Streptococcus pyogenes
A bacterium that causes infection, including strep throat, with an estimated 700 million infections and 160,000 deaths each year worldwide. In the nineteenth century, there were multiple observations that cancer was in remission for those infected with Streptococcus pyogenes.

survival benefit
The life-prolonging benefit of a treatment or medicine, sometimes expressed as the percentage of patients that survives during a given increment of time, often one year, three years, five years, or ten years, but often expressed in more complex terms.

Swiss cheese surgery
A surgery in which multiple lesions, up to twenty, are

removed from the liver, leaving the organ with the appearance of Swiss cheese. The removed pieces are regenerated by the liver. Developed in the 1980s by John Peter Minton.

systemic chemotherapy

Chemotherapy administered intravenously every three weeks or so over a period of time, sometimes more than six months. It takes about three weeks for the blood cell count to replenish sufficiently to tolerate the next dose of chemotherapy.

systemic overview

A formal review of a focused clinical question based on a comprehensive search strategy and a critical appraisal.

T cells

These cells, along with B cells and NK cells, are lymphocytes, and require B cells or NK cells to present antigens. There are various types of T cells, all of which mature in the thymus.

targeted therapy

A treatment in which the agent(s) are looking for specific targets, such as molecules expressed on the surface of a cell. Targeted therapy, in cases where it has been developed, is thought to create less "collateral damage" than traditional chemotherapy, in which rapidly dividing cells are killed but killed indiscriminately.

therapeutic intent

A phrase that differentiates a procedure or medicine that provides benefit to the patient from one that has some other purpose, such as finding out how quickly a person metabolizes a new drug. Medicare and insurance companies require that a treatment have therapeutic intent before they will pay for it. In many Phase I trials, where a small number of patients are used, the pharmaceutical companies generally pay for the treatment.

tissue microarray

A tool used by pathologists to isolate multiple samples of a tissue for testing. Separate tests can be used, for example, in identifying the cancer and in determining the rate of metastasis (how quickly the cancer is dividing). The ultimate goal is to help determine treatment and prognosis.

tomograph   A machine for making an X-ray of a selected plane of the body. For example one could get a horizontal view of the abdominal cavity with a tomograph but not with a normal X-ray. From the Greek for "cutting."

tomography   See tomograph.

total parenteral nutrition   See TPN.

TPN   Total parenteral nutrition. In some cases cancer survivors cannot eat, and their nutritional requirements are supplied intravenously through a device similar to a port. Nutrition is supplied during sleeping hours, leaving the recipient mobile during the day and even allowing the recipient to travel. Recipients of TPN can live for years afterward.

tumor

(Also spelled "tumour" and also referred to as a "neoplasm.") An uncontrolled or abnormal growth of cells, often first recognized by swelling. Some tumors are benign, no longer growing, and considered harmless. Other tumors are cancerous, malignant, and potentially dangerous, necessitating a treatment plan.

tumorigenesis

The progression by which normal cells evolve into cancer cells, involving multiple steps. The term dates to the mid-1940s.

tumor marker

One of at least thirty-eight substances, usually found in the blood or other discharge or tissue when cancer is present; however, there are other reasons these markers arise, so they are often only an indication of cancer. For example CA-125 (an antigen) and GCDFP-15 (a protein) are both ovarian cancer markers, but either can indicate a different cancer as well, or no cancer at all. Testing for cancer markers is a screening, not a diagnostic tool.

urologist

Someone who studies the clinical and surgical aspects of the urinary tract in females and the genitourinary tract in males. The term dates from the mideighteenth century.

urology

The branch of medicine concerned with the study and treatment of diseases of the urogenital tract (the urinary tract in females and the genitourinary tract in males), which includes urinary tract infection, the passing of kidney stones, kidney failure, and urinary incontinence, and other disorders. Coined in the late sixteenth century.

Venodyne

The brand name of the DVT compression system used during surgery that is expected to last more than forty-five minutes at Mercy Hospital in Baltimore, designed to help deter deep venous thrombosis, blood clots that could prove fatal. There are other compression systems that are commercially available.

white blood cells

See leukocytes. This term comes from Rudolph Virchow's 1847 German designation, *"weisses blut."*

X-ray

A graphic representation of what lies within the body; it is based on Wilhelm Röntgen's 1895 discovery. Today's CT scan is based on the same principle, though a computer reconstructs several X-rays. Röntgen himself suggested the variable X.

About the Author

Ebb Galvin is a teacher who has published articles in the fields of human interest, business, and air traffic control in small-circulation magazines. He also has written literary analyses of Anton Chekhov's *The Little Trilogy* and Juan Goytisolo's *Duelo en el Paraiso*. He earned his BA from Saint Bonaventure University in Olean, New York. He lives with his wife Lisa in Baltimore and has a talented son, Danny Galvin, who is an aspiring writer and comedic performer.

A portion of all author royalties for *Mercy* goes toward cancer research.